No E

'Becky is an incredible woman and we could all learn something from her attitude to life, and to living.'
Siobhan Sinnerton ITV Productions

'She's remarkably brave and her positive attitude is inspirational.'
Radio Times

'Breathtakingly courageous and honest. Her humour shines through.'
New! Magazine

'The story of how Becky has faced every woman's worst nightmare is a testament to the strength of the human spirit.'
Tessa Cunningham, The Daily Mail

'Becky shares her remarkable story with touching honesty and a lot of laughter.'
Lorraine Kelly GMTV

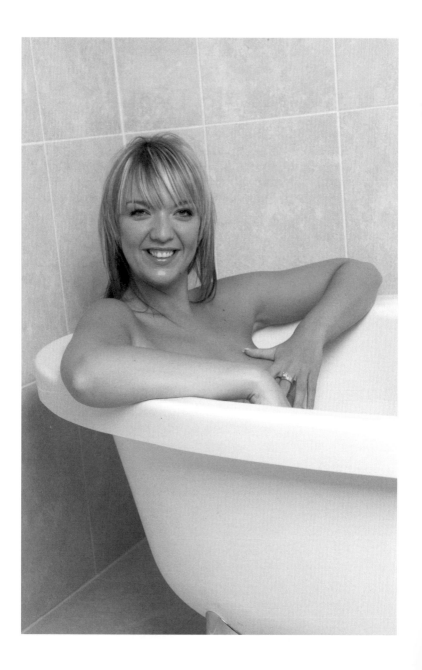

No Big Deal

'My breasts or my life' –
beating cancer before it happens

Becky Measures
with
Simon Towers

Medavia

Medavia Publishing
An imprint of Boltneck Publications Limited
WestPoint, 78 Queens Road, Clifton, Bristol BS8 1QX

www.boltneck.com

This edition published by Medavia Publishing 2006

A CIP catalogue of this book is available from the British Library

ISBN 0 9546399 3 6
ISBN 97809546399 3 8

Typeset in $10\frac{1}{2}$/12pt Palatino by
Academic and Technical Typesetting, Bristol
Printed and bound by The Bath Press

Cover design by Mark Ralph ATT & Clive Birch © 2006

CONTENTS

Foreword by Lester Barr 7

Preface by Professor D. Gareth Evans 8

Introduction by Becky Measures 9

It's My Life 11

Do, not Die 25

1780 and all that 41

The Bloody C 57

Me and my Mum 71

No Big Deal 89

What's it all about? 113

Genesis 127

The Big Picture 139

Tomorrow 153

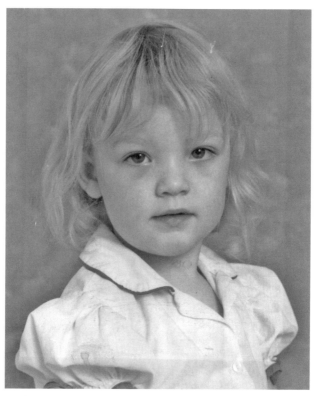

The age of innocence - three years old and at playschool

FOREWORD

by Lester Barr, Chairman, The Genesis Appeal

This book tells the story of two remarkable women – a mother and daughter – who discovered a dreadful truth about their family history. Most of their female relatives had died of breast cancer. Faced with this depressing information Wendy and Becky could easily have buried their heads in the sand, resigned themselves to their fate, or wallowed in self-pity or bitterness. Instead, they worked through some tough choices and came out the other side as two strong and remarkable women.

Together they have helped hundreds of others through the National Hereditary Breast Cancer Helpline, which they have established, and through championing the Genesis Appeal, a charity working towards breast cancer prevention for the next generation. The work they have done is incredible in turning a negative experience into a positive and having the bravery to help others in a similar situation. Theirs is the story of how two ordinary women can make an impact on the world through determination, courage and a desire to care for and help others.

PREFACE

by Professor D. Gareth Evans

Rebecca Measures is, like her mother Wendy, a remarkable woman. They have both had to deal with the spectre of hereditary breast cancer and have not been afraid to deal with this in the spotlight of media fascination. The way we look at one of the biggest killers in the world has been changed by the bravery of these two women. No longer do women have to fear the constant threat of breast cancer if they carry a high-risk gene such as BRCA1, but they know there is a real and not so frightening alternative. They have both shown that with or without the best reconstructive surgery a woman can feel confident and womanly. They are an example for us all.

INTRODUCTION

by Becky Measures

After the documentary for ITV, I managed to piece together a huge network of support, both socially and professionally, and they have all helped me get through this experience. One of the reasons for agreeing to do this book was to highlight how much of a part they all had to play in helping me, from friends and workmates to Andy and Gareth in Manchester. It was important for me to be able to tell my story, and to give an insight into how other people can make a difference in dealing with and overcoming the problems of one person.

One thing that struck me has been the number of people who have told me that they have found courage through my experience. It's not only been people facing what I have had to deal with, but others who have been forced to overcome hurdles, and that made me realise what a big influence my own mother was on me. It was made easier for me to have been brought up by a woman who dealt with the same issues, and it is my hope that other people will find it easier to approach their own circumstances, albeit in a different way.

My main hope is that people who have similar fears to me know that there are options available to them. They can see how I've coped with the decision, that there is a lot of support out there and that the medical world has moved on so much. I don't think I've done anything spectacular, I've not saved a life, I don't pretend to be anything other than somebody who has taken control of their own life, but if other people can take strength and inspiration from what I've done, then I'll know that all the publicity, all the work with Genesis, the documentary and this book, will have been worthwhile.

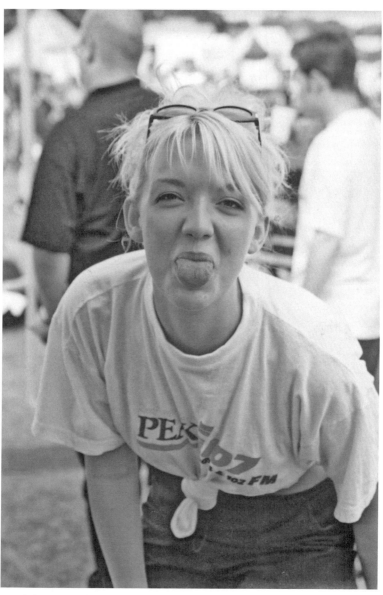

*Life begins all the time, so let's enjoy it – first job with Peak FM as a
promotional girl, here at Sheffield Show*

IT'S MY LIFE

'I knew that if I waited much longer my life would be at risk. Inside I felt fine, but there was something wrong that had killed other women in my family and I did not want it to kill me. It felt like there was only one thing I could do to stop it happening to me, because to me there was no other choice. It was obvious to me that I had to have my breasts removed or I could die.'

It is a situation that would terrify most 24-year-old women. Becky Measures is a radio presenter from Bakewell who was faced with one of the most difficult decisions imaginable. She opted to have surgery to remove her breasts of her own free will, despite there being no illness, no accident suffered and no physical ailment apparent to anyone. From a medical point of view her personal history was unblemished and the operation was not recommended or offered to her by a doctor or surgeon. It was a choice made of her own volition. It left many people shocked. A choice that attracted a lot of media attention, including TV appearances and an hour-long documentary, which aired on ITV1 in June 2006. People wanted to know why such a young woman, who had a successful career and no trace of illness, would willingly want to have her breasts cut off. Her story is one of courage, determination and the willingness to face disturbing facts by making shattering life-changing decisions that most women dare not contemplate. It also swam against the tide of known medical research, changing opinions and altering the approach being taken against one of the world's biggest killers of women.

Becky was co-presenting the breakfast show on Peak FM, a radio station in Chesterfield, when she announced to an astonished audience of more than 100,000 listeners what she intended to do. Her decision would shock and inspire a nation but none more than those closest to her.

'She was my little baby and I was worried about her', explained her father, Jeremy. 'I had a bypass two years before so I knew what big operations were about. She may have been well into her twenties but she was my little baby and age never changes that, you never want to think of anybody in that position let alone your own flesh and blood. My only consolation was that she was in the best hands because this was something that had come about through years of talking and planning. She was getting the best treatment anyone would get but of course you worry. In a major operation anything can go wrong. Like any father thinking about their little girl in surgery, you worry.'

'It was worse than going through it myself', recalled her mother, Wendy. 'I was so relieved when she came round from

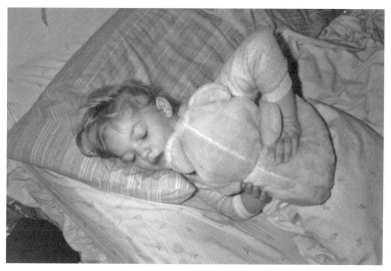

Caring, sharing: four-year-old Becky with her Care Bear

the operation. There is always concern when you see your daughter go through an experience like that. It was something that she felt she had to do and I believe she made the right decision for her.'

Becky was born on 13 October 1981 at Derby City Hospital. Wendy and Jeremy had been married for a couple of years and the birth of Becky was the defining moment of their life together up to that point. They had no reason to suspect at the time, but the chain of events that would lead to their daughter going under the surgeon's knife on 26 January 2006 had already begun.

Becky led a relatively normal childhood. In her early years she was unaware that her mother harboured concerns about her own future health, fears that had been with her for more than 15 years. It was something that did not initially affect a very young Becky, who shared her mother's interest in horse riding and had the good fortune to be given her own pony on her second birthday. She grew up on horseback and became a competent rider, winning a variety of showjumping awards as a child during the time they lived in Long Eaton, a small town not far from Nottingham. She also enjoyed her mother's love of theatre, taking up singing and acting before she had reached double figures. Even in her formative years she enjoyed the limelight and was never afraid of being the centre of attention.

When Becky was just 7 years old her parents split up. Jeremy and Wendy went their separate ways and Becky lived with her mother, still seeing her father at the weekends.

'You hear people say how they were badly affected by the break up of their parents but I cannot honestly say that was the case for me. Obviously I was upset, but we never really did much as a family before so in one sense not a great deal had changed. I saw my dad every week and most of the time before they split up was spent with my mum because we shared the same interests. I was always involved in what my mum did, whether it was singing, dancing or the horses.'

Becky was aware that her mother paid regular visits to the doctor. Her grandma had died of breast cancer at a fairly young age, leaving Wendy terrified at the prospect of getting the disease herself. Wendy's grandmother had also been diagnosed with breast cancer, although she was able to beat it, raising concerns that she could also be in danger. In 1990 they moved to a farm at Arbor Low near Monyash in Derbyshire, a move that would reveal the truth about her legacy. A chance meeting with lost relatives revealed that more members of Wendy's family had suffered and died from breast cancer than was first thought. It was time for her to make a decision.

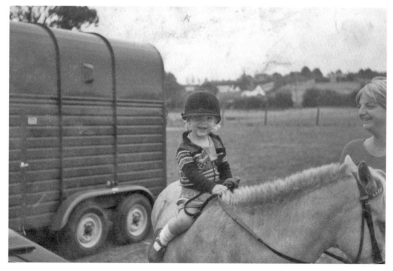

The first pony - Becky at two with Marigold

Wendy became convinced that this disease was targeting her family. Her concerns as a teenager that this may be a hereditary condition became more focused, despite numerous GPs telling her otherwise. She decided that she wanted to pre-empt this disease by having a double mastectomy, a course of action that baffled the medical world. Becky began to appreciate the extent of the problem that faced her mother and the lengths that she was willing to go to stop them surfacing.

'I explained to Becky that I was not ill and I was making sure that I would never become ill. I thought the best way to let her know what was going on was to lay it bare, so I simply told her I did not want to die. I don't think it came as a massive shock to her because we had talked about it before and she was very grown up for her age. It would have done no good at all to keep her in the dark about it, she would have only found out from somebody else, possibly in a way not to my liking. This way she could hear it from someone we both trusted.'

'Mum told me she was making sure that she would be OK in the future', recalled Becky. 'There was no sit down, mother to daughter moment or any big chats, I knew what had happened to my grandma and great-grandma but probably never fully understood the way I do now. It was no secret and everybody in Bakewell knew about what she was doing, Chris, my stepdad, helped me to better understand it. I was just told it was something she had to do.'

Becky also knew about breast cancer through her father's side. His mother had suffered badly from the disease and also had throat and ovarian cancer, so the presence of this disease was not a surprise to Becky. Breast cancer is a problem that affects roughly one woman in every ten. It is usually a disease that hits later in life but in extreme cases it can hit in the twenties and, in some very extreme cases, occur in teenagers.

The disease is diagnosed when DNA in the breast tissue cells is altered in some way and they begin to grow out of control. This uncontrolled growth forms tumours and they impact and invade organs. Unless it is caught and treated in time it can prove fatal. Symptoms can include a lump or swelling in the breast, a change in size or even discomfort and swelling in the upper arm. The good news is that only 1 in 40 people who go to their GPs with concerns over symptoms are diagnosed with cancer; however, once diagnosed a third of those die. It is a serious disease and once detected, surgery is the only reliable known cure and it is almost impossible to prevent.

'If you are talking about lung cancer, that is much easier to prevent', explains Lester Barr, a breast-cancer surgeon and chairman of a cancer charity geared towards prevention. 'Lung cancer is very much linked to smoking, so if you can stop people smoking, you can stop most people getting it. With breast cancer it is more complex. There are lots of things working together, including factors that are genetic. There may be dietary issues to do with the Western diet and lifestyle, because it is much more prevalent here than in places like Japan and China. Various chemicals in our environment could be playing a part as well. There are hormonal issues such as the Pill and HRT, pills we are using that may have side effects, and then there is the whole issue of improving early diagnosis, developing better scanning techniques to detect the early signs of cancer.'

The treatment of breast cancer is a big concern. Once surgery has been carried out there are extensive and intensive therapies to ensure the cancer does not return. Chemotherapy and radiotherapy are the most well known courses. Chemotherapy in particular can be a harsh treatment that poisons and results in debilitating effects within the human body. There are also less well-know courses such as gene therapy and immunotherapy that have varying degrees of success. The best form of defence against breast cancer for most women is early detection; that is why mammograms are offered to all women between the ages of 50 and 65 every three years. Unfortunately, it is no longer a disease that only affects post-menopausal women, it can strike much younger than that; however, though a mammogram is not recommended for people under 30 it is still the best method of early detection.

'The problem is the breast tissue is so dense in your twenties', explains Professor Gareth Evans, Professor of Medical Genetics and Cancer Epidemiology and a consultant at St Mary's Hospital, Manchester. 'It is very difficult to actually see anything in a mammogram, let alone pick up a cancer at that age. You have to use larger doses of radiation and that would increase the risk for the future of getting breast cancer, if you were using large doses as young as in your twenties. It is a combination of those two factors that means that the Government has said that we should not be using mammography screening under the age of 30.'

'The mammogram was the worst part of the run up to the operation', explained Becky. 'They put your breasts into this vice-like machine that crushes them vertically and then horizontally to get the mammogram images. It was absolutely agonising and I kept telling them that my boobs were too small for what they were doing. I could see the nurses looking at the image scans and frowning, that caused me concern and I wanted to know what the matter was. They told me there was nothing to worry about but that did not stop me becoming anxious every time the post came through the door, in case the results came back and showed I already had cancer.'

Becky had reason to be concerned. Her family has a history of breast cancer that has seen 14 confirmed cases throughout the generations; a statistic that forced Wendy to believe that she would be next. Watching her mother go through with a double mastectomy to avoid its effects was a powerful experience for Becky, who was 11 at the time. She understood what was happening and even at that age she was becoming image conscious and displayed an ability to deal with tough situations such as she was soon to face.

'I was always well developed when I was young. I started my periods at a very early age and had boobs from when I was about 9, but I hated them because I was a bit of a tomboy at that age, strange as it may seem now. I wore big baggy T-shirts and I did not like that part of my body anyway. I was the only girl in my year that had breasts, it was only when I got to the age of about 15 that it started to bother me because they had not grown anymore and everybody else's had.'

Wendy had grown up associating her breasts with death. She had them cut off because that part of her body gave her no pleasure and represented a threat to her life she did not want to remain. Becky had no such worries but still went on to become the youngest woman in the country to have an elective

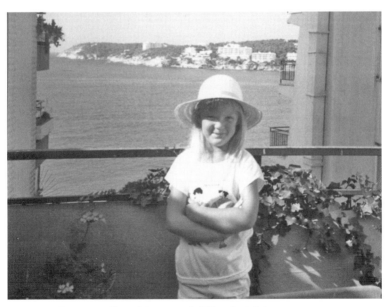

A sunny disposition - on holiday in Majorca at seven

double mastectomy. Wendy's experience gained media attention through newspaper articles and radio appearances culminating in a TV documentary that aired on Channel 4 in 1996. It helped raise an issue about breast cancer that goes some way to explaining Becky's decision. Wendy's concerns about the disease coming for her proved well founded. There was something wrong within her family that predisposed them to breast cancer.

'I saw Wendy in 1992', recalled Professor Evans, 'and she explained to me that she had initially gone to her GP in the 1980s and had been dismissed. Her concerns about family history were disregarded and she was told not to worry about breast cancer just because her mother and grandmother got it. When she came to me it was immediately clear that the pattern she described, the way breast cancer had affected her family, it had to hereditary. It was not consistent with chance and although shared environment could perhaps explain a couple of sisters developing cancer or even three, it would not explain the pattern over many generations that had affected her family. It was clear it fitted in with described patterns in the literature and that there really had to be a tendency.'

Breast cancer can be hereditary. Becky knew her mother's concerns and they were confirmed after scientists in the United States discovered a gene fault that can stop the body's defences dealing with the disease. If Wendy had it then Becky was at risk. It was a tough situation but not one that Becky had to deal with alone. Wendy's search for answers had led to a widened family network, all of whom were in the same boat, all having to face up to the possibility that they could have this deadly gene fault. The decision was never as simple as cutting off the breasts to remove the risk; there were people around Becky who were a huge influence. Friends, family and work colleagues were to play a major part in influencing the final outcome. There is no doubting the courage Becky displayed even coping with the choices she had to make, but people influence people.

First of all there is Becky's mother. She had already undergone a double mastectomy to stave off this horrific disease and campaigned to raise awareness of her situation. Her efforts altered the way doctors, surgeons and even scientific researchers viewed breast cancer and the way it should be treated. She had the power and the knowledge that would become so important to Becky, but she also had the parental responsibility to consider how and when to let her daughter know about a future that could include breast cancer. Having lived with the fear of this disease since the age of 16, she was stuck with the dilemma of having to tell Becky what was happening, but also having to protect her from being afraid for herself.

'I think I handled it correctly and put in the same situation again I would not change a thing. Not everybody agreed with the way I approached matters but it has made her the person she is and I think I helped her prepare for that day in the operating room. It is not something I wish to promote because not everybody could cope with that as a solution, but I think I did a damned good job of bringing her up. I am immensely proud of her, what she has done and how she handled it.'

Then there is Carl, Becky's boyfriend. They began seeing each other when she was 18, a full six years before the operation. How he dealt with any decision regarding her breasts, so often an integral part of any physical coupling, would affect their relationship and possibly Becky's decision. Carl would see Becky at her most vulnerable; become a confidant during moments when doubt might creep into her mind. There would be times when the gravity of the situation would become too much for Becky and how he reacted could be a vital apart of her approach to the operation.

'It probably got to him more than he let on to me. He would tell me that he had spoken to his mates about it and his friends have been good because they would ask him what was going on. He was just 27 years old when I had the operation, so he is still a young lad and part of a group of young lads, and it was nice to know young men could talk about it openly and be alright about it.'

Her work as co-presenter of the 'Sean & Becky at Breakfast' show on Peak FM was an important tool. Becky decided to go public with her story and broadcast the news of her decision to all the listeners across North Derbyshire. It allowed her to continue raising awareness of a situation her mother had made

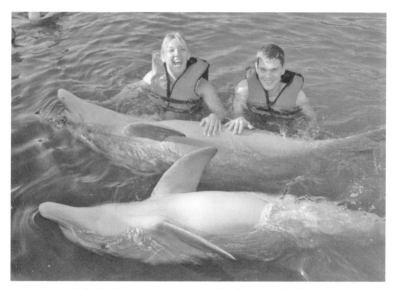

Cuba 2005: in preparation – Becky and Carl Price

public ten years earlier; it would also open up a part of her life that many women would want to remain private. It would invite messages of praise but also accusations that she was going through with the surgery in an effort to further her career. The pros and cons of baring her soul would be lived through the glare of the media and through a film crew that wanted to document the major developments. It would provide her with the opportunity to talk through her experiences and allow humour to enter into the equation with the banter between her and her co-presenter, Sean Goldsmith, likened to a brother and sister act.

'The whole thing was played out as though she was my sister and it is weird that although she has undoubtedly been through an awful lot, it never really hit home because to me it was just Becky. It still has not sunk in what a big thing it is she has done. People phone in and say she was so brave but to me it is just the way she is. I struggle to see beyond her being my colleague, friend and the bubbly person she is. To me it is strange because of how she has treated it; she never gave the impression that it was such a big thing. I think inside it was very emotional for her and it was a big thing but she never showed it off on the outside, possibly to her friends a bit more. I picked up on how she regarded it and that was how it always came across.'

Becky's cousin, Helen Cauldwell, was perhaps the biggest single influence. They became close after Wendy's search led to a reunion with other family members. Helen's dealing with the killer gene was a direct factor in Becky becoming the youngest woman to undergo her type of surgery. She also inspired Becky's attitude to the decision, making her realise that this genetic mutation was a ticking time bomb but need not be a death sentence. Without Helen, Becky may still be making up her mind and the outcome could have been devastating.

'What happened to me put the pressure on Becky to do something about it but she had to proceed in her own time. I think for some people it is so easy but it's about not putting your head in the sand and saying you will do something later. It was something that she needed to move on, but only when she was ready herself. What was right for me might not be right for someone else and the same goes for people who may have thought they knew the best for me. I think she made the best possible choices. I really hoped she would have the operation before she got any kind of cancer, so she did not have to go through it.'

Professor Gareth Evans became a close family friend. He was the one man who took Wendy's concerns seriously and the effect of that was to revolutionise surgical thinking towards breast cancer. His research and the findings of his team paved the way for Becky to use the science behind the discovery of a genetic fault. The technology to detect the ticking time bomb could be used to diffuse it before the clock stopped ticking. He helped pioneer a way of beating cancer that was based on prevention rather than cure.

'Becky was pretty much convinced that she had the faulty gene and had probably made her mind up about the operation before she was certain of the fact. It would probably have been more difficult for me to convince her that she did not have it because of what had happened throughout her life. She pretty much decided what her course of action would be before she knew the result. It might have been difficult to unplug from that knowing that she still had a population risk of breast cancer. Even though that was far less, her concerns may well have remained.'

The operation to remove her breasts is not complicated but it is severe. The procedure would take three hours with a further hour for the initial reconstruction but it is not without its risks. There are dangers with all surgical tasks that involve anaesthetic, although these are low with statistics suggesting one in every 200,000 people die as a consequence of the anaesthetic. There is also the risk of infection and scarring, or that excessive bleeding could lead to problems, although this is also rare. The surgeon must be sure to remove as much of the breast tissue as possible, any cells that remain are still at risk due to the genetic fault. The choice for Becky was whether the risks and any concerns over body image outweighed the fear of getting breast cancer.

The operation required a lot of careful consideration. It involved bringing the chest muscle forward, which would be used as padding before a series of expansions could be performed over a certain period of time. This would be used to make room for the implants that needed to be inserted in a separate operation six months later. The recovery time would be two months and Becky was prepared for the worst; if the reconstruction did not look as good as she hoped then she was ready for it. Once the reconstruction and the operation were performed, there would be no going back. Her decision would be absolute.

Most people would describe Becky as a very outgoing girl. Her career within radio was made possible by her determination to break into the media world she caught a glimpse of through her mother's documentary. She is very image conscious, a factor that makes her decision all the more remarkable, and enjoys a night on the town with her friends in Chesterfield. She has helped raise money for The Genesis Appeal, a cancer charity, and works with her mother to help make people aware of what breast cancer can do. If anybody knows the crippling effects this disease can have on people and their closest friends and family, it is Becky.

'I did not want to die and that was the beginning and the end of it. I thought long and hard about it, considered everything and knew that there could be a chance that I might never even get this blasted disease. I just could not live with the thought that I could get it, even though everybody is at risk. Like my mum I had to do something to put those fears out of my head and surgery was the only option. If people thought I was mad for having my breasts removed then that was their problem not mine. People could not understand it unless I gave them the whole story behind my decision, after that they got it. I would rather be walking about without boobs than six feet under with boobs.'

Becky never asked anybody to feel sorry for her. She accepted what was happening to her without apportioning blame to anybody, instead embracing it as an opportunity. She adopted the attitude that you have to make the best of a bad situation, and at times the situation became just that, because she was the only one that could change what was happening. She was not alone in dealing with it; her family had lived with this curse for generations and helped mould the system that would see Becky through this. There were opportunities to help other people whilst helping herself.

'How can I complain? Everything that has happened to me has made me the person I am today. I'm fit and healthy, there is physically nothing wrong with me, I have a wonderful boyfriend, great family and friends and a career that I have always wanted. It has not been an easy journey, but I might not have the same outlook on life that I have now if I had not gone through the bad times.'

'That gene is a part of me and part of my daughter', Wendy contends, 'and I would not change that. If you take away that part of her then her personality could be different, she might not be as tall, she may not have the confidence she has always had. It is just as much a part of her as everything else and I would never change anything so why should I want to change that. I am so proud of Becky and always have been.'

Eight generations and 14 confirmed cases of breast cancer. Becky's story goes back more than 200 years, long before science was able to determine what a person may die of long before they even know they are ill. Her story is all about choice and control, having those things taken away from her only to wrestle them back and seize the power of her own destiny. It was not just a question of life or death; the factors behind her life choices go well beyond something as simple as that. It came about from a lifetime of outside influences, medical research, historical background and personal tragedy. Becky gave herself the chance to live without fear, but the price would be high. She had found that living with a death sentence was no way to live.

DO, NOT DIE

It was the death of Becky's grandma that led to her eventual decision; it was not a direct inspiration. Becky had not been born when her grandma died at the age of just 43, but the way her mother Wendy reacted to it set the scene for the incredible decisions they would both face. Wendy was only 16 when her mother was taken by the disease that would shape the way she lived the rest of her life. However, apart from experiencing the kind of grief that would greet any daughter under the same circumstances, there was another concern that encouraged Wendy to find out why her mother died. It was not the first time breast cancer had revealed itself to her family and she wanted to know if she would be next.

Wendy's grandma had battled breast cancer and won before succumbing to the effects of ovarian cancer. This caused Wendy some distress, not only because two close female relatives had encountered the disease, but also because of the relatively young age it struck them; breast cancer was perceived to be a problem in the latter stages of life. It prompted the teenage Wendy to investigate further, concerned it might be more than mere coincidence, a concern not shared by the medical world.

'I went to my GP and asked if it could possibly be hereditary, in other words could I be at risk of getting breast cancer, and he told me there was absolutely no chance. He did not seem to understand my concern that I could be at an increased risk, that my chances of getting it could be affected by my mum and grandma. He seemed to believe the opposite was true, that because it had struck two generations earlier that it reduced the risk of my being affected. I was not entirely reassured but thought I would take it on board and didn't think it would kick in until my forties at the earliest.

'Over the next 20 years it was forever at the back of my mind but I never let it spoil my life, although whenever I went to a GP I used to ask if breast cancer was hereditary and each one used to tell me the same thing. In a way I was probably reassured by

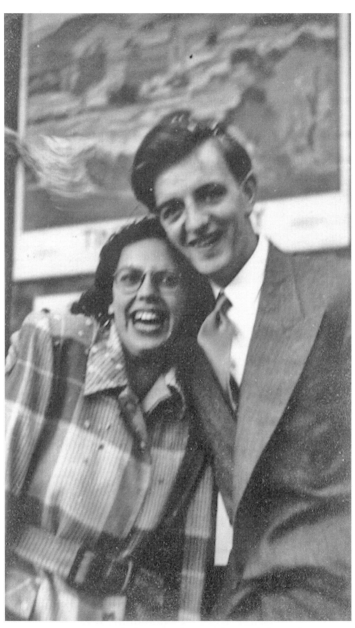

The genetic link – grandma, and grandad Land

what they said at the time because I wanted to be put at ease. I think I knew deep down that what they were saying was not true but, not knowing any better, it was more a case of hearing what I wanted to hear.'

Wendy never truly felt at ease with this assessment. She felt there was an ominous pattern that could only end with an inevitable battle against the thing that killed her mother. The medical world seemed unwilling to listen to her concerns so life went on with the fear that it could strike at any time never too far from her mind.

Wendy met and married Jeremy Measures, with whom she had a bouncing baby girl by the name of Becky on 13 October 1981; however things didn't work out with Jeremy and they separated before Becky's eighth birthday. She met Chris Watson in 1988 through their passion for showjumping and after a two-year romance they married on 17 March 1990. It was around this time that Wendy moved from Long Eaton on the Nottinghamshire border to Arbor Low near Monyash in Derbyshire. The move brought her closer to the answers she was looking for and it was there that she made her first startling discovery.

'I met up with one of my mum's cousin's daughters, Jennifer Cauldwell, and she told me that she had suffered from breast cancer twice, once at the age of 32 and then again at 39. Her sister had died at 38 and her mother had gone on to develop it in her sixties and she also had a cousin who developed it at the age of 48. When I told her that my mum and grandma had both suffered from breast cancer she could not believe it, it was then that we realised the true significance of its presence in the family. I knew there and then that what I suspected as a teenager was nailed on, that despite the fact that nobody had ever discovered it, it must be hereditary.'

The number of breast cancer cases in her family had jumped from two to seven across just six people. The doubts came back stronger than ever and Wendy gained a renewed determination to make the GPs who had dismissed her theories sit up and take notice. She went to the village doctor, more concerned than she was as a teenager and fully appreciating the consequences of her fears. Her husband Chris, who was aware of Wendy's unsuccessful fight to be heard by GPs on previous occasions, was surprised at the outcome.

'We came from the Nottingham area where the GPs were prepared to just dismiss Wendy's fears as paranoia, brushing off the prevalence of breast cancer as coincidence, but up here a little village doctor by the name of Graham Hurst not only listened to her but acted on it. He seemed more enlightened or at least more sympathetic to her concerns. It never felt strange that all of a sudden someone took notice of what Wendy was saying; it was part of the natural progression of her determination.'

'I wasn't particularly angry at what I had been told before', Wendy added. 'I didn't think the other GPs were being neglectful. They were just acting on information they believed to be true at the time and had never been confronted with this sort of query or situation before. Of course there were other families like mine, but I was concerned that there must be

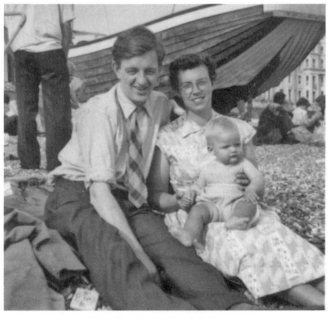

Fond family – Wendy with her parents

something wrong with my family. Dr Hurst recognised our family history and told me the important thing is that we catch it before it spreads.'

Something still did not sit right with Wendy. She was approaching the age when breast cancer struck her mother and the fears it would also kill her had grown. It was agreed that Wendy would be checked every three months and an early course of mammography was suggested. This course of action frightened her as much as the thought of cancer; there was a sense she was simply waiting for this deadly disease to catch up with her. It eased none of the fears she had harboured for more than 20 years and, if anything, it seemed that things had become more intense.

'I went for this quarterly check up and, though the doctor was a very earnest gentleman, he used to frighten me to death by looking over his glasses, feeling away, and he would suddenly stop. My heart would go into my mouth, wondering what he'd found. Of course he never found anything and it was elating to be given the all clear, but a month before having to go back the anxiety would return. There was just this feeling that I was gaining a stay of execution each time, it was not what I had in mind.

'After the first couple of occasions of doing this I thought to myself this was just preposterous, waiting to develop breast cancer and then hoping to catch it in time. I wondered if there were any drug prevention treatments, if early chemotherapy was an option and if I started to take it at the very early stages, would that be prevention. It felt like I was the only person who had prior knowledge that I was going to get something and I was just sat there waiting for it to happen instead of doing something to stop it.'

There was no way to determine if and when it would strike. It couldn't be prevented so, for the time being at least, the world of medicine was providing no answers. After all those years of her theories falling on deaf ears, her situation had barely improved. Wendy began thinking outside of the box and put an idea to her sister while they were out walking, as much in jest than out of serious thought. Perhaps if there were no breasts at all, the cancer would have nowhere to develop.

'I said, almost flippantly, "Do you know I've got a mind to just go and have these blasted things removed now, then I know I've caught it in time." It was the only decent idea I had come up with and it was said as a joke. There was no big thought process behind it, just an idle quip, but it made sense because it was not the operation that I was afraid of, in fact I was expecting to have to go through with it at some point anyway. What I was afraid of was enduring endless chemotherapy with the uncertainty of whether I was going to live and the subsequent worry that it could return.'

It was a suggestion that found favour with her husband.

'I had no qualms about Wendy's idea whatsoever and was asked about it quite a lot at the time because it was virtually unique. By then of course we had got the results of the investigation into the family history and it was blatantly obvious to me that the rules of evidence pointed to the fact that sooner or later she was going to get it or at least be extraordinarily lucky not to. As far as I was concerned, if she was happy having the surgery I was right behind it.'

It was a radical idea that provoked a response. It instigated an emotional reaction in people, as much down to Wendy's apparent calmness as to the procedure itself. Friends and family found it difficult dealing with the idea that a perfectly healthy woman could have both breasts removed to prevent a disease that may not even become manifest. It may have shocked people initially, but they still displayed a morbid interest in what she had planned.

'People told me how drastic it all was. I always told them that it was nowhere near as drastic as dying, but in the weeks leading up to the operation it always took at least 20 minutes for me to explain to people the full extent of the family history and the reasons surrounding my decision. Everybody wanted to know why. They had to understand what I was doing. I actually found myself cheering up everyone else by telling people that I was just going into hospital to remove the part of me where breast cancer developed. It was not about curing anything but preventing it. People just could not handle the realities of my decision unless I made them feel better about it. I was completely at ease with the situation and my husband was as well, it was everybody else that struggled with it.'

Wendy had battled for years for someone to take her seriously. Here was a disease that kills a third of those that contract it and her family had a familiarity with it that was a little more than disturbing. She had won that crusade, but asking them to perform such an outlandish procedure when there was nothing physically wrong with her was another thing. It felt like the conflict would have to be fought all over again; there was no way she was willing to wait to die. With past experiences of doctors not listening to her fears about a genetic link still strong in the memory, her hopes were not high. But life in Derbyshire was about to deal her another winning hand.

'I told the doctor I wanted the mastectomy now, to prevent breast cancer from ever happening, spreading and killing me. He didn't think I'd gone bonkers, in fact it was quite the opposite. He realised I had an appalling family history and that logic, not blind panic, had brought me to this conclusion. I realised it seemed extremely bizarre to the average conservative Briton, but to me at that time it was the most sensible solution. He agreed to send me to a surgeon and told me he had no idea what would happen after that, but for me the important thing was that he had listened and sent me.'

This would prove to be groundbreaking work but the surgeon took more convincing. It was one thing operating on somebody who was seriously ill with cancer but quite another operating before it had even appeared. This was not a procedure that was common and more groundwork was necessary. Wendy had been looking for treatments or procedures that could prevent cancer developing, while trying to come up with a way to prevent her playing the waiting game. There was nothing quite that advanced, but there was a research project that had been set up that would prove to be of mutual benefit.

Wendy was told about a family history clinic in Manchester that was looking for families with a history of breast cancer as part of a project to establish a possible genetic link to the disease. For Wendy this was another major breakthrough and marked the first time she had been told by anybody in the medical profession that, not only could breast cancer be hereditary, but also that research was being done to try and prove it. It was also when she met the man who would change her life and become a close personal friend, Professor Gareth Evans.

'I went with my husband to see Professor Gareth Evans and it was like a breath of fresh air. I expected him to argue against my decision because if everyone else thought I had gone bananas, then a man of science would take the same view. He thought that what I was proposing was reasonably sensible and accepted it as such. He pointed out quite plainly some of the down sides of the procedure from a physical and psychological perspective, but I never got the impression that he was trying to talk me out of it or looking at me as though I was overreacting.'

That meeting would change the way breast cancer was researched. There was nobody more appropriate to deal with Wendy's concerns than Professor Evans. He works as a consultant in medical genetics at The Christie and St Mary's Hospital in Manchester and specialises in the inherited predisposition to cancer. He also investigates rare and inherited cancer syndromes and associations of cancer that also run in the family. In terms of case studies, Professor Evans had found his woman.

'We were trying to find families like Wendy's to obtain blood samples to do what we call a linkage analysis and try to narrow down the location of the gene BRCA1 on chromosome 17, the one we believed could be responsible for genetic links to cancer. The more families you have and the more blood samples from multiple family members, the more likely it is you will be able to find the appropriate crossovers on the chromosome and be able to localise the gene. We contributed to the worldwide effort and Wendy's family was one of those that helped pioneer that.

'I challenged Wendy about her plans to go through with preventive surgery in a non-confrontational way, explaining to her that two or three years down the line there may be a genetic test that could reveal she did not have the genetic fault. I asked whether she would then feel she had made the right decision if the surgery had already been done. I also told her that eventually there may be better means of treating and curing or even preventing these cancers, but I could not give a timescale on that. Wendy was adamant she did not want to wait two or three years. If she got cancer in that time period she would never forgive herself. She had made her decision. I did not patronise her by telling her that what she was proposing was a good idea and to go ahead with it, I put some challenges in to make sure she knew all the facts about what she would be putting herself through.'

Carrying the gene would mean an 80 to 85 per cent chance of getting breast cancer. There was a 50 per cent chance of carrying the faulty gene and research already carried out suggested she almost certainly did. Wendy did not need to hear much more and Professor Evans was left in little doubt about what her decision would be.

'It was uncommon at the time but certainly not unheard of for operations to be carried out before breast cancer appeared. Wendy made it very clear that was her option; she did not want to carry on with regular screening and the doubts over how effective screening actually was. The very clear agenda of that meeting was that Wendy most definitely wanted to opt for surgery. She had thought it through over a number of years before meeting me and come to that idea independently of reading anything or having it suggested it to her. She felt that it was the right option for her.'

For many women, losing their breasts is losing their femininity. They are a part of the body that has become increasingly sexualised, often accentuated by dress and fashion, even referred to as 'assets' in some sections of the press and fashion industry. To make the decision to have them removed, a woman would have to be sure and there was little counselling available at that time because the procedure had rarely been carried out. Professor Evans had outlined the concerns, the main one from his point of view being about Wendy's body image after the operation and how she would cope with having a physical part of herself cut off.

'I told them that as far I was concerned, I had a good chance of developing breast cancer and a fairly huge risk of dying, so if I could do something that buys me a bit more life then that was

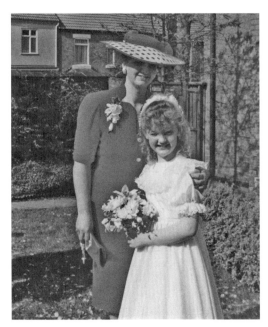

Wendy at her wedding to Chris, with Becky at eight

what I had to do. I was not concerned in the slightest about losing what could be a healthy pair of breasts; I wanted rid of the damn things that had caused me so much worry and so many problems within my family. There was absolutely no pleasure for me in that part of my body, just something that was there that could kill me.'

Any decision that affected Wendy in a physical way would also have an impact on Chris. He was as much a part of the consultation as Wendy, and the repercussions of how the operation would affect their relationship, both physically and mentally, were readily addressed. As with everything else they had confronted, Wendy had complete support from Chris.

'On a scale of one to ten in terms of grossness, it didn't even make number one. My attitude all the way through was that it was much better to have her here with a couple of bits missing than it was to not have her here, or watch her go through what was inevitable as far as we were concerned and get the disease.

The things I have seen in my time with the police, a couple of scars on your wife's chest were nothing to be afraid of.'

A revolutionary decision had been made. Staff at St Mary's Hospital in Manchester were left in no doubt that the operation would proceed and Professor Evans sent a letter to the surgeon outlining the case, but there were personal matters that also needed attending to. With a hectic workload on the farm, Wendy asked for a date in April 1993, the surgeons came back telling her she would go under the knife on 21 April. Despite her determination and insistence to go through with the operation, it was not enough to keep the nerves at bay.

'It was never about what I was going to look like or even the decision, it was the same feeling anybody would have going into an operation. I found it more important than ever that I should feel determined to go through with it; if I displayed any kind of reticence at all, they would stop the operation because it was groundbreaking stuff. That helped me because it gave me a built-in sense of having to be strong for everybody else as well. My main fear, first and foremost, was whether I would wake up, but that was certainly not enough to stop me going through with it. The repercussions of not proceeding were far more frightening.'

The operation was a complete success; Wendy was free from the shackles of breast cancer. Any fears that Wendy would suffer psychologically from losing part of her body were also allayed; her reaction was one of relief. After having worried about the onset of breast cancer and the possibility of leaving Becky without a mother, those concerns had literally disappeared overnight.

'I woke up the next morning and I felt the most privileged person in the world because I was in a ward with 29 other women, all of whom had been operated on for suspected cancer. They were all waiting to see if they needed chemotherapy, what their prognosis was, if it had spread, if it was cancer in the first place and I had nothing. They were all going for scans, waiting to see if it had spread to other parts of the body, for me it was just a couple of scars. How on earth could I feel anything other than very, very lucky compared to them? That was one time in my life when I felt overwhelming relief, like a huge part of my life that had been spoilt over the previous year or so since I found Jennifer and discovered the full extent of the family history was over. There were more important things to be getting on with, without worrying about the trivialities in life and that was what I did, I stopped worrying.'

Unfortunately the threat of cancer had not been eradicated. With the gene that Professor Evans had no doubt was present in Wendy and her family, there was still a significant chance of her developing ovarian cancer. She was brought in for a routine screening within a week of being released from hospital following the preventive surgery and the news was not good.

'They found an ovarian cyst and told me to come back in six weeks time to determine whether or not it was cancerous. You produce an egg from each ovary every month for reproductive purposes; you can have a follicle that is related to that. If it had altered during that time then it was just a follicle cyst because the other ovary is working, if it had not changed then it could be something more problematic.

'I was back a month and a half later, hoping it would not be the worst case of sod's law imaginable, and the cyst was still there. They said it looked OK but I was not willing to take the risk after going through the breast operation and decided to have my ovaries removed. My thought process was very similar to the one I went through in electing to have preventive surgery on my breasts. I told them that if I was in to have the operation then they could take them both out and have a full hysterectomy. I was 38 years old without any plans to have any more children, they could go out and get the biggest HRT implant they could find seeing as I had no risk of breast cancer.'

Wendy underwent a full hysterectomy only to discover that the cyst was benign. After two operations to stave off the risk of cancer, Wendy's time under the knife still was not over. There were more things to consider as a result of the initial operation, namely breast reconstruction. The surgery available was not as advanced as it is today and reconstructive surgery had to be done at a later date and booked six months in advance. Wendy and Chris had another decision to make, one that was no more straightforward but a little less severe.

'Having the reconstruction at the time of the operation would have meant they could not remove as much of the breast tissue, therefore the risk of getting breast cancer would remain. For me it would have been reduced but it would still have been there and my feeling was that if I was having the procedure, I wanted the risk reduced as much as possible. The idea was to have the reconstruction at a later date for a more successful preventive operation.

'I went back to see the surgeon and I could not decide which size they should be, so they sent me away again with three different-sized prosthetics. To this day the reconstruction still has not been done but it never really bothers me anymore. I do not need to wear a bra or any prosthetics and nobody seems to notice anymore, people have just got used to me. It's not that I was against reconstruction, just that I've not got round to it and it's not the most important procedure to me, although it is still a possibility for the future. I have always said never say never.'

Wendy became more involved with the family planning clinic. There was a growing sense that she could help women and families in her position avoid going through the battle she went through to get accepted. The memory of being turned away from GP after GP was still fresh in her mind and the evidence was mounting that there were other families in the same predicament. Whether or not they knew it was a different story. There was still plenty of work and other families to find to further the gene theories on which Professor Gareth Evans was working.

'I remember wondering how many people had been turned away like I was. Their lives could have been saved before the breast cancer had become critical. It was important to me that people knew that this fault was there and that other choices are available. At the very least I wanted to make sure people were aware that there were GPs sending people away that should not be sent away and subsequently have no idea they could be at risk.

'There was no media attention and I knew there was a serious danger that women in my position may not have been offered screening and died because it had not been detected in time. Bear in mind how I felt, it was like a huge burden had been lifted and I felt so free. Maybe it was worth telling my story somewhere so people knew there was another option other than waiting to deal with the disease, a choice that was nowhere near as horrific as the conclusion. That was when I decided to get in touch with a newspaper, to be helpful more than anything.'

Wendy's struggle to raise public awareness took a giant leap forwards when the *Independent* published an article in 1994 telling Wendy's story and Professor Evans' theory on genetics. It was intended to be a factual piece to outline alternative choices in preventing breast cancer and to make women aware that their family history could play a big part in the chance of developing the disease. Rather than becoming a one-off article, it opened the floodgates as the media world picked up on Wendy's story, a welcome intrusion for a family trying to raise awareness of new medical theory.

'A huge influx of television companies, magazines, newspapers, you name it, were all ringing up wanting to do various documentaries and interviews with me. It was great because the information that I wanted to get into the public domain was reaching a wider audience. I never expected anything quite like the level of interest it sparked off. People were just so astonished about what I was saying. It was a revelation to most of them.'

Not all the media coverage was positive. While most of it was factual and allowed the situation to speak for itself, some sections and editorials ridiculed Wendy and her family. There were accusations that they made decisions based on paranoia. Others were more condescending, insinuating that Wendy had ignored GPs who tried to be reassuring in pursuit of a medical expert who would agree with her. Then there were the publications that ignored the facts and concentrated on a different aspect of the decision and how the family coped with the situation; a form of journalism that aroused consternation in Wendy.

'I was unprepared for the silly publicity. I had plenty of magazine interviews, the first of which from *Bella* was so atrocious that I felt physically ill. I wanted to go out and buy up every copy so nobody could read it, it did not begin to convey the manner in which the interview had been given. It started off suggesting I was looking at a photograph of my mother with tears dripping down my cheeks and that is just not me at all. I would never say that even if it had happened that way, it was just so sentimental and never got close to approaching the real issue and that riled me up. I would rather there was no publicity at all than articles that over-dramatised it. It did not portray how I felt, I was elated rather than traumatised and it took the focus away from what was really important, trivialising it from something physical and potentially life saving to something emotional and that was wrong. For it to be worth anything it had to come over as a positive thing otherwise it is better off not knowing.'

Wendy faced some difficult questions. The interviews were coming thick and fast and her experiences and the decision made were laid bare for everyone to comment on. For her it was a necessary tool to prevent people from being turned away and falsely reassured; so, far from being an intrusion, the media attention was encouraged, but not all of it.

'From the moment I read the *Bella* piece I made the decision to ensure all the publicity was on my own terms. I had to have complete control of the copy to make sure there was no more sentimental drivel written about my family and me. As a consequence I loved doing live interviews because nobody could fiddle with things like that, they could ask any question they liked and I had an answer for all of them. I was quite lively about it and was told I gave a good interview. For me it was easy because I had nothing to hide and could easily answer everything. I loved the confrontational questions, my favourite being the one that criticised my decision, the one most interviewers thought would throw me. I ask tell them if they were faced with a 25 per cent chance of dying, wouldn't they try and do something about it?'

The support from her husband and family was unwavering. Chris was a big part of the decision and also had a part to play in the ensuing media circus, providing support when it was needed.

'The spotlight was not on me and rightly so. I had my job, which got me out of the house, so quite often I was out anyway.

The times when I was there I accepted they had a job to do and it took time. Questions have to be asked two or three times, the setting up often takes longer than the actual filming but I never had any trouble with it. Wendy always regarded it as an assistance to spread the word. She knew this was far more widespread than anyone had anticipated at the time. It took her a long time to get herself heard and the feeling was that if she could make it easier to get other people heard then it was necessary.

'The inaccuracies were the only real problem. It made us both very careful in terms of what we called the lower-class publications. They were just after a good melodramatic story and made sure that was what they got. The problem of course was that people reading it would have no idea that the scene did not play out like that and therein laid the problem. Wendy's decision to vet the copy was not out of arrogance, it was out of the need to get the right message across.'

A documentary was broadcast on Channel 4 on Tuesday 27 February 1996, detailing Wendy's story. It was an hour and a quarter-long programme that took on Wendy's reaction to her discovery of a family history steeped in breast cancer and her operation. It was initially proposed to be a journey through the decision making process and the subsequent attention, exposing the ways Wendy had helped change medical procedure and opinion. It would also take a close look at the genetic links, dipping into the research and taking a glimpse into what the future may hold for other families who suspect they might be in the same position. What the film crew got when they followed Wendy was a new research project that could potentially get to the heart of the gene fault and discover more people who had no idea they were at risk.

1780 AND ALL THAT

Wendy had conquered breast cancer in a way few had even thought of. Not only had she beaten her mother's killer, she had also persuaded the medical world to accept her way of thinking and ensure a procedure previously regarded as extreme was a viable course of action. For most women who had undergone such an emotionally and physically draining struggle, the temptation to relax and take life easy would be too great to resist. Wendy had spent the best part of 25 years worrying about breast cancer catching up with her, seemingly with nobody willing to listen. It was this factor that caused her to carry on fighting and push the boundaries further in an attempt to make others like her realise that there are alternatives to simply waiting for cancer to arrive. Wendy had got what she wanted, but the operation and decision still caused some exclamation and was not totally accepted. More work needed to be done and the media world still had a big part to play in making her story known.

Channel 4 approached Wendy with a proposition. They wanted to film a documentary about her trailblazing decision, operation and the subsequent genetic research to be called 'The Decision: Living in the Shadow'. It was to be promoted as a focus on one woman's remarkable story, how she dealt with the pioneering procedure and update the situation by delving into the research projects involving Professor Gareth Evans. Never in her wildest dreams did Wendy think her actions would become so important to warrant the attention that was coming her way, but it brought back vivid memories of previous experiences. Still a little cautious about a media keen to over-dramatise, she only agreed to co-operate after spending time with the producer. It proved to be a move that ended up saving another life and thrust Wendy and her family to the forefront of genetic research.

'Channel 4's concept for "The Decision" was originally to follow me and my reasons for having preventive surgery. It was so unknown at the time and nobody had even thought about doing it. Then I thought that maybe I should find out more about the rest of the family so I looked into the family tree. Originally, it was research based on helping Professor Evans find the gene, but once I got started it became more serious. As well as the research angle I got curious myself, and to put the number of hours in just for the fun of it you have to have an amount of interest or get paid. It is very time consuming but it has thrown up a number of curiosities and revealed one or two secrets.'

Having found a way to nullify the threat, the search was on for the source. Barriers had been broken and medical thinking turned on its head but there was still a need to understand exactly why this was happening to Wendy's family. Her search yielded some unexpectedly quick results. She discovered a woman by the name of Jean, not too far down the generational line, who had died at the age of 58, an age Wendy thought was relatively young. She sent off for her death certificate, which contained a piece of information that Wendy had half expected: this ancestor had succumbed to the familiar foe of breast cancer. For research purposes this was a major find because Wendy's grandmother and Jean's grandfather were brother and sister, meaning the gene had been passed down to her through the male side. It was a branch that was worth pursuing further.

Jean's husband, Harold Farnsworth, was the one who registered the death certificate. At the time he had worked as a college principal in Brighton, so the documentary crew followed Wendy through this line of enquiry. She wanted to know if this particular relative had a daughter, because if he had there could be a whole new family line at risk of the disease.

'I had to go and track this guy down but realised if he had been a shopkeeper it might have been a little more difficult; however, luck was on my side because Farnsworth was a relatively unusual surname. Directory Enquiries was no use because I had no idea where he lived and he was ex-directory in any case, so I set about ringing all the colleges and universities in the Brighton area until eventually I came up with one that remembered his name. The secretary said there was a Farnsworth who used to be the principal at that college but

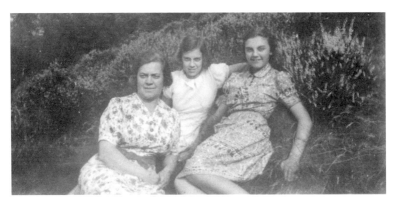

Generations – great aunt Lily, grandma Jean, and her sister, Betty

retired ten years ago. I explained the scenario, told her that his mum had died from breast cancer and that we have eight other cases in our family so it might be important to let them know in case he has any children.'

It was becoming ominously clear that the gene had far-reaching powers. The number of confirmed cancer cases within the family was rising as the search gained momentum. The

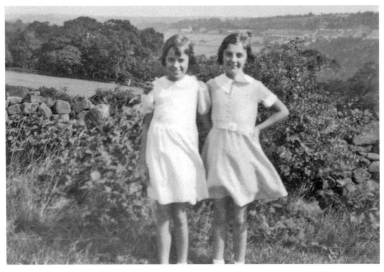

Grandma Jean and auntie Betty

problem was far more prevalent than Wendy first feared. However, the consequences in this case could prove more deadly. If they had had a daughter, the only family history they could possibly have known about was the single death of her mother. If she had harboured any concern similar to the one Wendy had over her own mother's death, it would have been dismissed because no pattern would have been discovered in such a small section of the family tree. Having explained the situation to the secretary who agreed to pass on her number, it was not long before Harold got back in touch.

'The secretary had not told him what it was about but it turned out he remembered my mum Jean, who had apparently been a bridesmaid at their wedding, but contact had been lost with the family after they moved down south. I told him I knew his wife had died from breast cancer and that there had been other cases in the family. I also told him that we knew it was down to a gene because a common linkage had been identified and we needed to know if he had any children. He had a daughter who was 42, so that was when I asked him if he felt she ought to know. I explained that she might wish to take the test, without suggesting she should rush out and do what I did, but at least find out if it was worth getting regular screening. I knew it was not my decision to make but thought I had to at least make him aware of a connection between our family and breast cancer that goes beyond coincidence.

'Within a few hours he rang me back and told me that he would get in touch with his daughter, Vanessa Smith, and explain the situation. It would be foolhardy to think that ignorance is bliss because he would never forgive himself if something happened to her and he had not passed on this information that could have warned her. That was when contact was made and I confirmed what her father had already told her. Her first reaction was that the whole thing was just bizarre. This relative had appeared out of the blue, one she had no idea existed, with the bombshell that she had a 50 per cent chance of developing breast cancer, maybe even more. It must have been a horrible phone call but it didn't seem to upset her.'

'Initially I thought it was hilarious', recalled Vanessa, who left Brighton in 1970 and now has a teenage daughter and a son of 16, whose future daughters could also be at risk. 'We just laughed because there were all these relatives that we never knew existed so we actually thought it was quite funny until the next day when we realised we had to confront this. Wendy had already seen Professor Evans at the family history clinic so I got the contact details and went along myself to get the ball rolling.'

Wendy was treading on dangerous ground. The situation with Vanessa, though comparable in terms of the physical situation, had a completely different shift when looked at from an emotional viewpoint. Breast cancer had been a part of Wendy's life since she was a teenager and she had lived knowing the possibility that it could strike at any time. Vanessa may not have made that connection. What right did she have to bring those fears to another person? Wendy had battled to such lengths in order to banish the disease from her life, but not everybody would have arrived at the same conclusion. If somebody had the same knowledge but could not face undergoing surgery, they could go through life wondering if and when cancer would take hold. The situation had thrown up an interesting moral dilemma for Wendy that she would have to confront before continuing her attempts at tracking down the origin of the gene.

'It could potentially save her life, but it could spoil it just as easily. To have this cloud hanging over her, knowledge she otherwise would not have had, would she struggle with the thought that she was at such a high risk of developing a disease that kills? A dilemma, but on balance my consideration was how I would feel if I had not made any effort at all to let her know, only to hear later down the line that she had been to the doctor about her family history, been told there wasn't one, maybe not even checked herself out and then developed breast cancer. I could not have lived with that so I felt it was absolutely the right thing to do and her father obviously did as well. She may well have cursed me at the time but hopefully in the future she would live to be pleased.'

On this occasion the concerns were unfounded. Vanessa decided that if breast cancer was going to hit her the way it did her mother, she wanted to know. Professor Evans told her there was likely to be a genetic test available, but not for another two or three years. There would be a tense wait for Vanessa who, unlike Wendy and Becky, was not armed with a lifetime of knowledge that breast cancer was a problem in the family. This was not the only thing Vanessa had to deal with that was new to her but familiar to them, Channel 4 was filming her.

'That actually helped because Sally Dixon, who was the producer, was so supportive, and part of the programme involved my husband and I talking about our feelings, sometimes together, sometimes separate. It helped because perhaps we would not have said so much had they not been there. I knew nothing about the family history, just that I had a 1 in 12 chance of getting breast cancer along with the rest of the female population, but I was never one to self examine that often, just very occasionally. I had to wait 18 months for the gene test to become available and, for me, that was the worst time. I think I had three mammograms in that time and they were clear but I had to know so that I could deal with it, that was why I went ahead with the test.'

Vanessa's link with the killer gene fault was confirmed, the test came back positive. Wendy's detective work had unearthed an incredible discovery; that a previously unknown family member, tracked down through a death certificate, had been found with the same tendency towards breast cancer. For the film crew it would provide a defining moment in genetic research that followed the path of a woman who had not only fought to make herself heard, but had begun to change the way cancer treatment and prevention was perceived, and carve open new research avenues. If Wendy could trace a family member through previous cases of the disease and death certificates there could be others out there. For Vanessa a big decision had to be made, one that only two years previously she never thought she would ever have to make.

'It was a shock but you have to take the bull by the horns and get on with it. I had been given the results and stayed awake all night thinking about it. By the time morning came I just told my husband, I was going to have the surgery. He was quite surprised and he thought it was a quick decision but it wasn't because it had been on my mind for 18 months. I knew what all

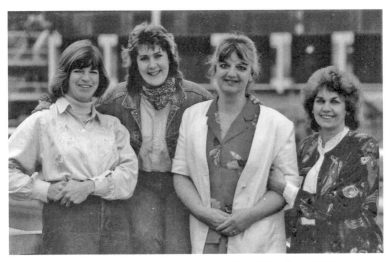

The long distance link – Helen, aunt Diane, Wendy and Vanessa

the options were and was just waiting for the test results, so once I had those it was obvious what had to be done. People were horrified at the suggestion of cutting off a healthy breast. People said that to my surgeon as well, horrified that he would even consider performing such an operation because it was so new. I was never against the idea of having the operation; I just did not want to make a decision until I had the facts. Once they had arrived, I knew I had to go through with the operation.'

An amazing chain of events had led to the same conclusion. Preventive surgery was taken as an option to obliterate the threat of a potentially deadly disease that had killed the mother of the woman in question. The first overwhelming factor of this outcome was that the form of defence Wendy had fought to make public had been taken. The second was that researching back through the family tree could potentially save lives by revealing a pattern of breast cancer that would otherwise have gone undetected. Wendy's persistence had been rewarded again through the discovery of another incredibly brave woman who was not afraid to confront the genetic flaw that she had inherited. Any future thoughts about divulging such information would have to be carefully considered, but it was an action that Vanessa embraced and was more than thankful for.

'If she had not got in touch I could be dead, it is as simple as that. My mother died a week off her 59th birthday and I'm not far off that now. Every woman needs to make up her own mind. What I did is not right for everyone and you have to look at it very carefully because there have been a few problems with the implants. I needed to go back to hospital to have them adjusted and they are the sort of things my daughter has to be aware of when she decides to confront it. She's going to university this year and has her whole life ahead of her and I don't want her bogged down with it right now. She needs to enjoy herself. The power to deal with it will still be there in five years time but she will have to start thinking about it then.'

The documentary appeared to move a nation. Wendy's attempt to reach people was beginning to bear fruit as she began to get a response from all sides, including women in her situation. Not only was the media frenzy in full swing, Wendy knew the programme had served its purpose when she began getting letters from members of the public. It seemed there were many other people who had experiences with breast cancer that led to fears for their own safety, fears that had not been heard until now.

'I had an awful lot of letters from other people who had found themselves in the same position. One particular letter that really touched me was from a young girl in the Nottinghamshire area who wrote ''Dear Mrs Watson, I hope you don't mind me writing to you but I feel that at last I've found someone who understands how I feel. My mum died when she was 27 from breast cancer, her mother died from breast cancer when she was 26. I am 25, I have a little girl of two and a half years old and the thought of a third generation growing up motherless has always filled me with terror. But the breast cancer clinic that I'm under, when I mentioned preventive surgery, won't even talk about it. They push me away and say don't be so silly, but I think it's the only thing available to me to be absolutely sure.'' '

Wendy had become an inspiration to hundreds. She had become the kind of person she was looking for when trying to confront her own anxieties all those years ago. What came out of this public response was the clear fact that many more families were afflicted with a deadly gene fault, similar to Wendy's, but had gone undetected. She had proved that by detecting a family pattern of breast cancer and tracing the lineage back, it was possible to follow the path of the gene and prevent it from having its intended effect. This line of research could potentially save lives. The way the work into gene theory was progressing, the requirement was there to go as far back in time as possible.

Wendy's nemesis had been discovered by the time filming had begun. The particular gene fault had been pinpointed as BRCA1; the very gene that Professor Evans had suspected was behind the growing number of breast cancer cases in Wendy's family. The first evidence of the gene was found in the United States in October 1990, not officially identified until 1994, but described in the kind of medical literature that detailed patterns of cancer over many generations. It was a vital breakthrough in the search for answers to Wendy's questions and Professor Evans needed more help from her.

The search for understanding was gathering pace. Wendy took it upon herself to find out how far back the gene fault went to see if it could shed any light on when and if it would strike Becky. It was at this point that the relationship with Professor Evans became more defined as their mutual interest in the research became inextricably linked.

Professor Gareth Evans started out in paediatrics before becoming involved in genetics. Initially his interest came as a consequence of looking at inherited conditions in children and recognising patterns of abnormalities. Over time it became clear that high-risk genetic conditions could also affect people later in life, manifesting itself in milder physical forms such as baldness or more severe illnesses, ailments and diseases such as heart disease and forms of cancer. He branched out into the latter part, specifically cancer, resulting in his eventual meeting with Wendy and a mutual interest in the nature of research available in tracing the gene and its source.

'I started doing genetics at the beginning of 1990 and it became clear to me immediately that a proportion of breast cancer was hereditary, but there were still sceptics in those days. Very frequently you would see letters from GPs and surgeons in 1990 and even up to the mid-1990s that were telling people to stop worrying and cancer was not hereditary. But there were some very good epidemiology studies and some papers showing there has to be a small component of even common cancers, like breast cancer, that were clearly hereditary and that there were genes being passed down the generations that were predisposed.

'We started offering the genetic test in April 1993 and the gene itself was not identified until October 1994. It was an exciting time and Wendy's was pretty much the first family in the world to be offered predictive testing. It was interesting to see what people's decisions would be, how people used the information and whether they chose to have the test at all.'

This interest manifested itself in Vanessa's situation. The success of finding her and the realisation that she had fended off the effects of the gene fault through their groundbreaking work was still fresh. Professor Evans' findings leant credence to Wendy's work tracing her ancestry and, combined with the positive start in delving into her past, more painstaking work had to be done to extend the tree back as far as possible. There was clearly a high concentration of the BRCA1 gene in her branch of the family, so a search for the source commenced. It was important to see if the gene originated from her great grandmother or great grandfather's side, especially in light of Vanessa's lineage.

'I started looking further into my family tree, widening it out and sending off for death certificates to try and find out where the gene had come from. Eventually I found my great-great-great-great-great-grandmother's death certificate that indicated she had died from breast cancer in 1849. It was an incredible find for me, not only because it proved that they were aware of breast cancer, but also because it was being documented in death certificates. Ovarian cancer was another matter, it would probably have got mixed up with other things because it was not easily diagnosed and there were one or two illnesses that didn't make sense. I have yet to discover any signs of ovarian cancer in the 1800s, which leads me to suspect that some were put down as something else.'

Wendy hit a brick wall at 1837. That was the year civil registration started in England, which meant there were no death certificates before that time. It was becoming increasingly problematic to find out more about certain sections of the family, it was also becoming difficult to extend the family tree back towards the present day. The tree was extended across to such an extent that it was a major task bringing it back to the present day, especially with records difficult to obtain.

'I have gone back a long way, I've widened it out and am in the process of coming back down to present day, to the descendants of all the people I have found. It is slightly more difficult because you have to go and find out who all these people are, many of whom have got married. The internet is a very useful tool when trying to find out things that go back hundreds of years because there are censuses available. You know that in a ten-year period if somebody is on one census and then not on the next then they have either died or got married. You cannot imagine looking through a whole lifetime, so it is more difficult coming back forwards and I have to think of a way of tackling that now.'

Historical documents are notorious for throwing up misinformation. However, modern-day census reports also create numerous problems because of the nature of 21st-century life. The most recent census threw up a list of a million people missing from the previous records that did not marry into a different name or die. People go on holiday, go travelling, fail to fill out the census correctly, they go missing in the post; there are lots of reasons why information can go unrecorded or fail to turn up on records. This was also the case 200 years ago, although the causes of the frustrations were different.

'You get thrown off by red herrings because you come across someone who appears to be missing. On one census a person may have put their name down as Mary Anne and on another it was Anne or another variation, those sorts of things happen quite frequently. Their ages get altered enormously, especially the ladies because you would find out that when they got married, they were younger than they should be. They told their husbands they were younger than they really were and slowly over the years their age would creep back to what it should be. How they got away with that amazes me but it happened a lot, which really threw me.'

The history lesson revealed one more intriguing piece of information. It involved Wendy's cousin Jennifer and her

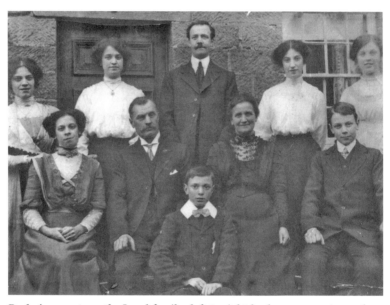

Becky's ancestors: the Land family; left to right:back row - great grandma, Ida, great uncle Tom, Nellie, May; centre – great aunt Lily, great great grandpa and his wife, Harry; front – Wilfred

daughter Helen, whose experience had such an effect on Becky. It was known that Jennifer's father, Rex Holmes, did not have the gene because he was tested as part of Professor Evans' research into the percentage chance of getting breast cancer and linkage patterns. What he did have was an unusual and unexpected connection to the family tree.

'His grandparents were cousins in our family who got married and produced children. Their son, Rex, married one of my great aunts, or maybe it was one of my mum's cousins, which is an incredible coincidence and may go some way to explaining why Jennifer and Helen got cancer so early in life. We thought he was nothing to do with the family at all, particularly as he did not carry the gene fault, but actually he has connections with two lots of the family because it was his great grandparents who were cousins. He could have introduced some element into the genetic make-up that made it worse for them, especially Jennifer who got it twice, although environmental factors cannot be ruled out. As an interesting sideline Rex developed cancer of the oesophagus. I found the whole discovery fascinating.'

Wendy resurrected the poser that fuelled many critics of gene theory. The question of how many cases in any family history are gene related and how many are due to external factors can never truly be determined. In 1992, around the time the research into linkage surrounding Wendy's family was being carried out, statistics showed 1 in 12 women would contract breast cancer in their lifetime in the UK, a large percentage when dealing with such a deadly disease. Professor Evans needed the history of families like Wendy's to establish just how these outside influences and the appearance of a gene fault could affect the chances of developing the disease.

'The first question to consider is what constitutes a lifetime and we approximate the lifetime expectancy of a woman to be 80 years of age. The current evidence is that if you look at an average "at risk" estimation of a woman developing breast cancer by the age of 80, it is approximately one in nine or ten within their lifetime. Even in this instance it varies based on geography; it is probably nearer one in ten in the north, but in the south it would be nearer one in nine because there is evidence to suggest that you get a difference based on socio-economic groups. The higher socio-economic groups have higher risks and it is often down to issues surrounding when you have your children, because the later you have children or if you never have children at all, the higher the risk. At least a substantial proportion of that difference is when people have children.

'In terms of risks, if you do not have a family history then your chance of contraction is nearer 1 in 12, but the risk could go up to as high as 80 to 85 per cent if you carry a fault in the BRCA1 or BRCA2 genes, but you can only prove that in a genetic test. The maximum risk we would give someone in the clinic was if they had a very substantial pattern like Wendy's on one side of the family. We would give them a 50 per cent chance of having the gene and then a 40 to 45 per cent chance of getting breast cancer in their lifetime. In Wendy's case we knew there was a gene fault, but the risk factor only goes up above 50 per cent if we know for sure that it is there.'

Wendy has barely scratched the surface of her voyage through time. The research has the potential to yield some incredible results but it is a mammoth task, far removed from the type of document that can be hung on the wall of your average landing. Wendy began the lineage on the reverse of a piece of wallpaper that now extends some 15 feet across. It has produced 14 confirmed cases of breast cancer with many more likely to be found once the tree is brought back into the present day. Wendy is also working on other family trees for the clinic and the work is still invaluable to Professor Evans.

'What we are very interested in looking at is how the incidents of breast and possibly ovarian cancer have changed over time, whether there has been a substantial increase over the last 100 years or so. We can potentially see generational changes in breast cancer incidents happening younger and younger in successive generations. Certainly from our preliminary data and other studies in Iceland and North America, it looks as though the risk of developing cancer at younger ages is virtually tripled so there is a very large increase indeed. Wendy's research is going to help find out how far back this goes.

'It is possible to potentially trace the originator of that particular mutation, what we call "The Founder". Some mutations have already been assessed as more than 3,000 years old, so if the mutation is that old there is little no chance of tracing it back. Some of these mutations are probably only 200 or 300 years old and as such they would be amenable to that sort of approach if we can go far enough back with the tracing in the family. There is one case where we have 11 families with the same BRCA2 mutation; we know they all occur on the same genetic background. If she could link all of those back to a single individual in history, you can be pretty sure that is the person who started it off.'

The earliest known carrier in Wendy's family, based on the linkage research from Professor Evans and Wendy's own detective work, is Elizabeth Land who was born in 1780. She died of breast cancer in 1849 but not before having a son who in turn had a son of his own. The gene was traced through a total of four lines of sons until it reached Evelyn Land, Wendy's grandmother. The gene was then passed onto Wendy's mother and to Wendy herself, the strand currently lies with Becky. From the single parentage of Tom and Annie Land who gave birth to Evelyn on New Year's Day 1887, the gene has been positively identified or supposed through linkage in 19 out of 37 descendents. All of these can be linked back to 1780, but Wendy does not appear convinced in her abilities to trace the tree back to a single carrier.

'You could never know the answer to that because the earliest breast cancer we know is Elizabeth, but where she got that from will remain a mystery unless I could test everybody in the Derbyshire region for our mutation. I would like to see that type of research that gets everybody who has a family history in the Derbyshire and Nottinghamshire area tested, to see if there is this mutation in other families because we would know they were related. Then I could do a family tree on all those people who have our fault and do it that way. That is a possibility at the moment, but what we are thinking of now is to try the other option of finding the relatives via the gene testing. Of course that depends on if people want to go through with the test. A dilemma I have already experienced when I tracked down Vanessa.'

There is a long way to go on this line of research but there were more pressing cases in the present day. Becky had yet to be affected in a direct way, apart from her family connection to the gene mutation. It was not that she was unaware of how breast cancer could affect her, more that she was still very young and had time to experience life before taking the gene test and thinking about the options available to her. But if Becky thought she had time, that comfort would soon be taken away from her. Her connection to the disease that had caused her mother so much concern and dominated her life for the last ten years was to rear its ugly head again. Becky was about have her first look at what breast cancer can really do.

THE BLOODY C

Breast cancer had cast a shadow over Becky from a very early age. It had killed her ancestors and she had witnessed her mother go through drastic and unprecedented surgery in order to avoid contracting the disease. The dangers associated with breast cancer were thrust to the fore in a way that few would be able to deal with at such a young age. Becky had made her mind up to take the gene test, but youth was on her side and she had yet to see first hand the damage this horrific disease can do and the pain inflicted by the treatment. A certain amount of complacency had set in regarding when the preventive surgery should be carried out, but this feeling was about to be shattered. The experience of another close family member would change Becky's perception of how to proceed in a way nothing else could.

Helen Cauldwell was one of the women who took the initial gene test with Wendy and discovered the chances of her getting breast cancer were high. Her blood relationship with Becky is fairly remote, Helen's mother Jennifer is Wendy's third cousin, but as the family tree revealed in Wendy's studies, the gene has passed across more distant generations. Despite this it is remarkable how similar they are, if not in looks then certainly in personality. Both have a confident nature and an endearing tendency to speak from the heart and open themselves up to people, a feature that saw the two develop a social relationship. They had become very close even before breast cancer had its influence.

Helen was only 17 when the chance meeting between Wendy and her mother Jennifer threw her life into a different direction. It was then that the full extent of the family gene was revealed in terms of confirmed cases of breast cancer and it was then that Helen learnt she could also have that very gene.

'It all came about at the same time', Helen recalls. 'It was Wendy who pushed to find the gene, being on the same generation line as my mum and close when they were younger.

My dad was telling her about my mum having breast cancer and of course Wendy's mum had died from it as well. She put all this information together and said, "right, what are you going to do? Someone has to do something." At the time they were looking to locate the fault. They knew there was one so they pulled our DNA to try and locate it. It was all quite exciting because meeting up again like that and finding the gene, it all happened at the same time. They thought our family was such a major player in the gene research.'

Cancer had struck Helen's family five times, killing one of them. Her mother beat the disease twice and her grandmother also had a brush with it and survived. Her mum's sister had lost her battle with a different form of cancer, but because she was only 38 when it struck, breast cancer may not have had time to develop. A little further down the lineage, Helen's grandma's sister was diagnosed, as was her grandma's brother's daughter. The condition had cut a swathe through the women in her family and Helen had to take the genetic test soon as possible. Becky was only 11 at the time but not too young to understand the implications of what was happening around her. Not wanting to shy away from the realities of the situation, she also wanted to get involved.

'I remember quite clearly we were all sat round the table at Moorhall Post Office, me, mum, Helen and her mum and dad and everyone had to give a blood sample. I recall being really gutted because everyone was giving blood except me because I was not old enough. Me and Helen went and played shop because everyone else was giving samples and sat around the table just talking, very bizarre to see.'

Helen was much less confrontational in her approach to breast cancer. Both she and Wendy had lived with its effect but whereas Wendy's mother was killed while she was a teenager, Helen's mother had beaten it, giving her an altogether different perspective on how to deal with it. Becky had found somebody else who had lived with the disease in a very similar way, both well aware of its immediate presence and how it would affect their futures. The way both had learnt to deal with the subject also drew parallels when it came to talking about how they coped with a family connection to the disease. Wendy confronted it head-on but Helen was also able to recount stories of how cancer was never a word to be whispered.

'It has always been very open in our family. The boobs are out all over the place. When my mum first had her operation she did not have any reconstruction, she had these prostheses that were like blancmanges. Well of course we used to steal them and put them on the dog's head, they would be lying about on the stairs, so it has always been a very approachable subject for us. It was such a serious thing that perhaps subconsciously we thought that it was always going to happen and we have got to make the best of it. Hopefully we succeeded in doing that.'

Helen decided that she had to be sure. She made the choice to take the genetic test in 1994 when she turned 21, and it confirmed that she did have the faulty gene. The fear she may have had about dealing with the consequences of knowing she was likely to follow in her mother's footsteps and contract the disease were realised. Helen took it all in her stride.

'It did not change my outlook on life at all because I knew the disease was there so it could not creep up on me, it was

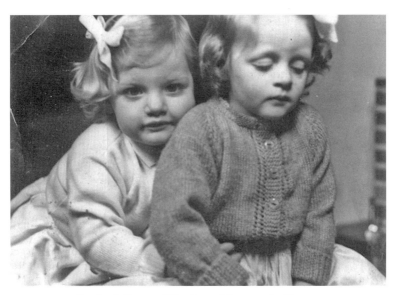

Good relations – Wendy and her cousin Sharon

something I had lived with. For example, some people live under the cloud of knowing heart disease runs in the family and this was no different. I was pretty sure that somewhere along the line I was going to have some sort of problem. It certainly helped that I was not the only one who took the test. Vanessa, Becky's Auntie Diane and Wendy all had it done at the same time because that was when it became available. It was good to have everyone around talking about it. Everybody was telling me I was doing the right thing because prevention is better than the cure, which it is.'

The clock was ticking. Despite the warning of numerous cancer cases in the family, she decided not to opt for surgery straight away. It was believed the risk was not serious until the early to mid-thirties and there was no evidence to suggest carrying the gene lead to such an early diagnosis. Rather than rush head-on into an operation that would still be available in ten years' time when the risk would be higher, it was a case of life goes on. Helen continued running golf clubs in Matlock and Bakewell as well as doing what most people do in their twenties, meeting people and fulfilling an engaging social life.

'It was very much a case of back to the old routine and the opportunities to have the operation just passed me by. There was always a reason not to go, such as preparing for the club's centenary year or simply because we were always very busy in general. My subconscious mind is a lot bigger than my thinking mind. There is not a lot of space in there, but there was a lot happening in the back telling me that I must get round to having it done. It was not a case of willingly putting it off because it was something I was afraid of, it was just that I never actually got round to doing it.'

Delaying would prove to have serious consequences. Her mother, who lived in Blackpool, was going for a screening in Manchester so Helen arranged to drive up to St Mary's Hospital and meet up for lunch just after her 29th birthday. Instead of biding her time in the waiting room, Helen decided to go and see Professor Evans for a conversation that may well have saved her life.

'You wait for hours in hospitals for everything and you are always hearing about new drugs and treatments so I went to see if there were any new trials happening in the near future. While we were chatting he told me that I should have a screening and booked me in for the following week to meet one of his colleagues. I went to the breast care clinic at The Nightingale Centre and the breast nurse said she would give me an examination. I thought I knew all about self-examination, but I was mistaken and did not realise the extent to which you had to stretch your body. She had me in all sorts of contorting positions with my arms up in the air, something nobody had actually told me. While doing the exam she found something and sent me off for a mammogram that confirmed there was definitely a lump.'

A week passed before the test results confirmed their worst fears. Helen had delayed surgery too long and breast cancer had returned to the family. The news would have left most people devastated. It was Professor Evans who broke the news.

'Gareth was upset because he had to tell me and my partner Pete, who was obviously very upset. It was a strange experience for me, you sort of go on autopilot. Despite knowing there was a very high risk of me developing cancer and knowing there was

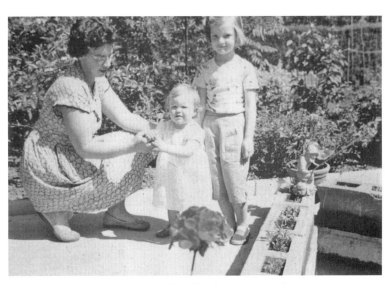

Aunt Diane with Wendy in the garden

a tumour, for it to come back positive was still a shock. Even though I knew it was going to happen, I was always under the impression it would affect me later on and I would have had surgery by then. I should have felt regret that I'd not had the operation but that was not the case. A decision had been made somewhere in my subconscious that I was waiting, but luckily we found the tumour before it had spread too far.

'Telling everybody was the next big step because nobody knew I was going to the hospital. People would casually ask if I was all right and I would end up telling them I had breast cancer. The reaction was usually hysterics, but I was confident it was all going to be taken care of and everything would be all right. It was a difficult thing to tell someone else because you have come to terms with it yourself but you know that other people will react in a certain way. You cannot keep it a secret and it was not something I wanted to hide, but the words had to be chosen carefully. Quite often you would think to yourself, "I didn't put that very well to that person so I have to tell these people a different way." It is hard to know exactly how to tell anyone, especially people close to you.

'I never look back and wonder if I had done something differently then this would not have happened, because I am quite a lazy person and I believe in fate. If anything I think it did better for Becky because it made her think that she needed to get a move on and get the test done to get things moving.'

The news had severe implications for Becky. She had yet to take the gene test because it was believed the risk at her age was minimal. The manner in which she was approaching the decision to take the test had parallels with Helen's approach to preventive surgery. Suddenly time was a factor and never could there be a more stark warning against the dangers of not acting on information than the situation Helen found herself in. There was an advancing sense that things were beginning to catch up with Becky in the way they had caught up with Helen.

'My life changed that day', Becky recalls when her mother Wendy gave her the news. 'As soon as I found out Helen had breast cancer it was just total and utter shock. She had taken the genetic test and as far as we were concerned it was not supposed to hit until the early to mid-thirties, so I could not believe it. As soon as that had sunk in and we'd asked if she was going to be all right and had gone through that period of concern and found out the next course of action for Helen, it suddenly dawned on me that I was going to have to get tested.'

For Helen there was no more waiting. The tumour had to be removed and the consensus was that it had been detected at an early enough stage, though it was still Stage Three Aggressive. Staff at St Mary's wasted no time in arranging a date for the operation. After an eight-year delay for the preventive surgery Helen had just a week to prepare for going under the surgeon's knife. The hectic social schedule and heavy workload that was such a factor in putting the procedure on the back burner ground to a halt in a fortnight. However, the swiftness of the situation proved to be a blessing.

'I was really pleased with how quickly everything moved because it did not give me a chance to worry about it. I was very lucky that I got in so quickly because as soon as it was detected the ball was rolling. One Friday I went in for the biopsy, the next one I went for the results, the Friday after that I went in for the pre-med where they take your blood pressure for the anaesthetic and it was all very much a roll on.

'My outlook to contracting the disease was positive. My mum had it twice and recovered fantastically, my grandma as well so in my view it is not necessarily a killer even though that is often how it is perceived, something very final and associated with death. Wendy was in a totally different situation when she made her decision because her mother and grandmother had died, so she had a different perspective to me. I knew it was well within me to beat this thing and hopefully we had got to the cancer as quickly as we could have done, which was a great relief.'

The mastectomy and reconstruction was a success, but the real horror story had yet to unfold. There was to be extensive and intensive after care and treatment, coupled with the anxiety that it may have spread or even return, as was the case with Jennifer. Part of the reason Wendy made her radical decision was to avoid the after effects of an operation to remove a tumour. The battle had been moved away from the surgeons at Wythenshawe Hospital and would resume at The Christie; on this occasion there was no family member with whom she could relate the experience.

'I think I must be a pioneer', Helen remarked, almost with a sense of pride. 'My grandma had to have radiotherapy but my mum did not have anything, no drugs, chemo, radiotherapy or anything. It was not as bad as it could have been. The ward I was on was a really special place because all the women in our bay were all having the treatment at different stages; it was like some sort of club. Due to the fact some of us smoked, we used to get out of bed first and go for what seemed like a mental self-help group session amongst ourselves. We were in a hospital, all being treated for cancer, all sat outside next to the mortuary of all places, smoking! We were all wandering about with drain bags and drips, it was quite unreal, like something out of a 'Little Britain' sketch. Not that I would advocate smoking by any means, but it did put us together in a group because we had that in common, that was a really interesting experience.

'The nurses were fantastic as well, really kind, and that made it so much easier. The food was rubbish of course. I know everybody says that about hospital food but this was the worse I had ever experienced in a hospital before. All my friends and family had to call at Marks & Spencers or McDonald's before visiting to get goody bags for me. A friend of mine from Tideswell, who likes a glass of wine as much as me brought two flasks, one full of chilled white wine and the other full of red. We would sit and have a bit of a celebration that I had come through the op, eat sausage rolls and drink wine through straws in flasks. That was a nice part of it, kind of like being back at school or university.'

The treatment meant more than just a decline in her physical health. Life-changing decisions had to be made to aid Helen's recovery. The requirement for a less rigorous working timetable began to hit home as the need to eat, sleep and recover properly between treatments became paramount. She stepped down from running Matlock Golf Club, while Pete retrained for a job that kept more regular hours to better support her during the ordeal. Friends became more important than ever and they rallied round, helping her move house from Matlock to Bakewell, decorating and allowing her to concentrate on recovering. Her outlook on what was happening remained positive, but when recounting her time trying to cope with the treatment, Helen remembered just one feeling above all others.

'Being sick! All my hair fell out during chemotherapy, which was quite exciting for a while, a very different look for me. There were quite a few interesting wigs, but I never quite got the hang of tying the bandanas. I had my chemo at The Christie Hospital, which is a specialist cancer hospital in Manchester and they were marvellous. I had different people taking me to hospital every three weeks who had no idea what chemo was like. It shocked a few people who were seeing it for the first time. It is a vile experience, you are basically poisoning your body and it kills the cancer, but you are being poisoned as well. My body knew where it was going when I was driving to the hospital so I was starting to be sick in the car on the way.'

This gave Becky a first look at the disease that caused her family so much pain. The realisation was beginning to set in for her of just how serious the situation was becoming for Helen as she began a course of chemotherapy. Her health was more at risk due to the nature of the treatment, she was more susceptible to infection and fatigue as her physical appearance also began to change and her body reacted to the different drugs that needed to be used.

'I had a combination of three different drugs that was referred to as FEC, an acronym of the drugs involved. It is a common one used for treating breast cancer and I had it fed intravenously through the back of my hand. Because they were putting needles in all the time, my veins collapsed so they had to move it into my arm but those veins collapsed as well. It was extremely intensive because your body has got no antibodies and the risk of getting any type of infection is very high so you have to be careful about what you eat. If you get any type of temperature you have to go to hospital, you really have to look after yourself.

'Even now I can still taste it, it got into my system, into my mouth. They had foot-long syringes on the table and you know that they are going to be inserted into your body. The three drugs all did different things and there was one of them called Epirubicin that made my bum sting because it hit the nerve ends. I had the strangest sensation as the needle went into my arm because it was my bottom that was feeling the pain. All the juices were going into my body, the needles going into my arms and hands, I was throwing up and my backside was in agony. It was difficult to know exactly how to react to all of that except that it really was not pleasant. I can look back on it now and laugh because recounting it makes it sound so absurd, but that was chemotherapy.'

The poisonous nature of chemotherapy brought further complications. Her health began to deteriorate further as Helen eventually succumbed to the more extreme nature of the treatment. Her veins collapsed and the doctors had to put in what they call a Hickman Line. It was a procedure that put her life still further at risk.

'The drugs burnt through my veins so they had to put in a tube that went through my chest, just below the neck to go straight into the blood supply. This was where they could take the blood out and inject whatever they had to into my system. Because they had put a foreign body into my system that had a two-way flow, the risk of infection was even higher and a lot of care and attention had to be taken to reduce that risk. It needed flushing through every week so the district nurse had to come and see me on a regular basis. This was very dangerous for me and I did develop an infection of the breast, I was riddled, but you had to keep on smiling to get yourself through it. They were trying to find the veins that had collapsed, but the Hickman Line was so infected they could not get it in, so they had to take the line out. They cut a hole in the skin to get the line in, like a piece of thick hosepipe dangling out. That was the area that got infected. It was very serious at one point but thankfully I pulled through.

'I had to deal with other things going on around me as well. A friend of mine called John died after becoming very poorly with pneumonia. Another friend, Richard, went through two courses of chemo and the cancer had returned. He said he was not having the treatment again, he didn't want to go through it, which a lot of people thought was strange. He died and everybody wondered how he could just give up like that, but once you have experienced it you can understand why people decline any more treatment. The process only involved little bits at a time but I would not like to go through it again, however, if I had to I would.'

It took six months before she was free of chemotherapy, just before her 30th birthday. Her friends threw her a surprise party as a joint celebration, to mark the completion of chemo and a landmark birthday. It had been a while since she was able to enjoy a night out, taking in Bakewell, Lady Manners School where Helen had been a pupil, then on to Chatsworth and back to her old school where friends and relatives waited with champagne and canapés. The night was an important part of the recovery process, marking the completion of what many feel is the hardest part to endure. There was good reason to celebrate; however, the trial was still not over.

'I started radiotherapy in September, not long after my 30th birthday, which was an altogether different experience. Rather than make me ill, this just left me tired, although there was plenty going on to keep me occupied. I had "Tonight With Trevor MacDonald" filming my radiotherapy, which was happening at Weston Park in Sheffield. I turned up at the wrong hospital at one point, went up to reception with a full film crew to tell them I was there for my radiotherapy and they just looked at me blankly and said "We don't do that here." I just had to turn round to the crew and say "Sorry, we seem to have the wrong place." It was an easy mistake to make because I was going to the Wythenshawe for surgery, the Withington Hospital for clinic and The Christie and St Mary's in Manchester as well. At least it lightened the atmosphere and kept it fun, which suited me fine.'

Becky was forced into a year-long wait after finding out Helen had cancer before she was able to take her genetic test. The wait was not intentional, there are lots of implications to consider before taking the test that revolve around life insurance. Even if the test comes back negative, it puts a person in a higher insurance bracket; the reason being a person must think they are at risk to take the test in the first place. Once all this was in place, the test could be taken.

'You have to go through appointment after appointment before they let you do these things', Becky explained. 'You have to have all kinds of assessments to make sure that you know the implications. Helen was a huge support to me even though she was going through her own thing at the time. I knew I had to have the test anyway; it was just a case of when. I was always going to leave it until my late twenties because it seemed that there was no rush, or I would just do the same as Helen and go to have it done when I had the time or had to make a trip up to Manchester. You really do think you have so much time with no sense of your own mortality, which might seem a little strange coming from a family with such a background and a history of breast cancer.'

Helen had to go under the knife once again. A partial reconstruction had been done at the time the tumour was removed, but a full reconstruction still had to be carried out. She had a date with the surgeon again on the 3 March 2003 and it proved to be a more complicated matter than simply taking out the implants and inserting the silicone.

'They had to cut me open again where they had taken the breast tissue, they had to remove the nipples as well because the cancer can potentially return through them. They needed to take as much of the tissue out as they could, I also wanted as much of the cells removed as possible so they took my lymph nodes as well. They often do that for people who have had breast cancer because that is the first place that it spreads to. You have about 15 under your arm and the cancer had spread to three of them. As opposed to it being a solid block, they had begun to break away and that was why I had to have the radiotherapy and the chemo. The last part of the reconstruction involved tattooing nipples onto my breasts, purely for cosmetic reasons, but they look pretty good and now all my friends have got tattoos. All of this was a breeze compared to chemotherapy.'

The risk of a recurrence never truly disappears. Once cancer has struck a percentage risk always remains and that is one of the major reasons behind many decisions to opt for preventive surgery. Helen hopes to have made a full recovery, although doctors say if you have been clear for five years then that is a healthy sign and Helen has just entered the fourth of those five years. Even though the disease is no longer being treated to such an extent, the after effects are still being felt.

'My cancer was oestrogen fed, so they switched my oestrogen production off by giving me some injections into my stomach, putting me through a premature menopause. Nobody knows how long I should remain on this medication; everybody has a different take on it. The last time we spoke I was going to stay on it for three years and see if my ovaries came back on, so that if I wanted kids I could have a little time bracket to do that. After that I could have a hysterectomy but cannot have HRT because that would be putting the hormones back in. That is what they are trying to block.

'Another thing about waiting to have the surgery is that if I do want children, I would have to have them quickly and that should never be the reason for having kids. If I was going to start a family it would have to be because the time was right, not because the time was available, but if I put it off too long I lose the opportunity altogether. That is something I do feel bitter about and when I wish I had done things differently.'

Helen has faced every hurdle throughout this experience head-on but she does respond when anyone suggests it was down to her being positive.

'It helped me and I like it that people can see that quality in me, but it is not a very pleasant thing to hear for the relatives of those that have died. It was never a conscious decision on my part; it was just how it happened for me. I feel bad for those that have died; they did not all lose the fight for the lack of a positive attitude so there is much more to it than that. It is always a double-sided thing for me and cancer has never been such a frightening word because of its familiarity. Cancer is still referred to cautiously as the Big C, almost like a death sentence or a word that people find difficult to say out loud, whereas in our family it has always been talked about very openly. In a roundabout way having it in the family helped me cope with it better.

'I wish the surgery had been performed sooner, but as for feeling bitter about it, no way, because this is my path. I can't change it so I don't dwell on it. None of us have got hindsight so there is no point wishing you did because that is what will drive us all mad. I dealt with what has happened so I don't dwell on what hasn't, you cannot live your life based on what ifs. People I know and have got to know have died through cancer, so it is very easy to see that it can take your life. I never take life very seriously any more, you are here for a very short time and going through this type of experience only makes that more obvious.'

Becky could no longer view her future health with such certainty. The age barrier had been dropped into the twenties and the risk of waiting too long had proved to be one not worth taking. Everything was set for Becky to take the test and act on the information, but how did watching Helen go through a year of recovery affect the decision she had to make about her own life?

'As soon as I found out she had cancer I decided to have the genetic test, although I knew it would come back positive. The thing that sticks out most in my mind about what happened to Helen in that year was something she said to me; word for word it went like this, "I feel that this has happened to save you, and if I had to do it again, then I would." I was taken aback that someone could be so unselfish. What she said implied that she would go through all that a second time, amazing, but that is Helen all over. There was never any question of what my decision would be if the genetic test came back positive. I knew what I had to do.'

ME AND MY MUM

Becky had seen the debilitating effects of breast cancer first hand. It hit Helen hard, but the consequences could have been far more severe if the disease had not been found so early. The operation would have been more difficult, the treatment more severe and the pain level much more difficult to bear. Helen would have gone through all of that without the guarantee of recovery and the threat of a relapse would always have hung over her. Becky had no other choice but to take the genetic test and act on the information given, she owed it to herself and to Helen. With the option of waiting to have preventive surgery now out of the picture, the consequences of a positive test would be to remove a pair of healthy breasts, or gamble with the chances of waiting to contract the disease. Wendy found it an easy decision having watched her mother die, Becky had no such negative image but had her own reasons for the life choices she was about to make.

Becky had been always been aware of her mother's obsession with breast cancer. It may not have been related to fear but the facts were always simmering in the background, brought to the boil every few months when Wendy went for a screening. Wendy's decision not to pull the wool over Becky's eyes in terms of what could lie ahead served as ample preparation for future events and she had her reasons for exposing her to the truth at an early age. Wendy never had the choice of knowledge when she was young; her GPs did not take her concerns seriously, but the feelings of doubt she had in their attitude stayed in the back of her mind. It gave her the view later in life that she would have slept better at night if she could have known earlier. It was with the benefit of hindsight that Wendy decided to raise Becky with the philosophy that knowledge is power.

'What I was more concerned about was that I knew about breast cancer when I was 16 years old and I was worried about what happened to my mum. I wanted to talk about it, but when

I went to the doctors or spoke to anyone about it they always seemed to think that I did not need to worry about it. They wanted to shut me up more or less, which effectively closed the door to the things I wanted to know more about. What it did not do was stop me from worrying. I certainly wanted Becky to experience things differently. Children can worry about illness more than anything else so it seemed a good idea to have these things in the open. As things were revealed to me I told her as best I could. I never kept it a secret because from experience it was not the right thing to do and I think I handled it the right way.'

'I never really remembered mum worrying about it', Becky recalls about her time growing up. 'She was never that type of person. She was always a happy-go-lucky person in my eyes; one minute she would be doing one thing, the next she would be doing something else. Her worries, if there were any, were never inflicted on me because that was how she dealt with things. She didn't want to get upset in front of me so that is not the way I remember things happening.'

Children can be stronger than parents like to believe. There is a temptation to wrap them up in cotton wool to prevent them from growing up too soon and ensure they never come to harm. Wendy had reason to think the disease she feared would come for her might also lie in Becky's future and she needed to be made aware. An early explanation that would normalise the situation could help prevent it from becoming a drama in the future. Besides which, Becky was growing up fast.

'I thought she was very capable as a child. She was always tall for her age so people treated her as though she was older than she actually was. She was incredibly tall and her feet were the same size as they are now when she was 9 years old. She mixed with older people as well because of the kind of socialising we did back then. I used to take her to the showjumping where she would mix with girls who were older than her peer group quite happily. She was a lively child who was good fun, never found things difficult and was not difficult herself. She took most things in her stride so explaining things to her was never a problem.'

The little girl was forced to grow up fast. They moved from Long Eaton to Arbor Low and that was when things motored forwards in terms of Becky's education. Wendy learnt more about the family history and believed the threat she had inherited from her mother was also there for Becky. Wendy had laid the groundwork, but far from being a frightening experience finding out more about her ancestry was yielding a different emotion in her 11-year-old daughter.

'I remember it being exciting, sitting down with family members I never knew I had. It was amazing for me at the farm, our nearest neighbours were half a mile away, then all of a sudden you go three miles down the road and there were a load of relatives I had never met. It was a different world for me really. I got to meet people they knew and experienced different things. We even bought the shop from David and Jennifer and moved in there, so that was another big change in my life. Of course it was at this point that I met Helen, who was to play such an important part in the future. It was like one big adventure.'

But the adventure had a serious side. Whether Becky realised it at the time or not, the reunion was what led to the realisation that breast cancer was going to be a fact of life within her family. Wendy's decision to have preventive surgery was taken when Becky was approaching her teenage years. At that age the worst most girls have to worry about are spots, puberty or boys; trivial matters compared to what Becky had to deal with. Her mother was going in for major surgery of the kind that had rarely been performed before and this despite no hint of breast cancer. As far as teen angst goes, this was as hard as it gets.

'I was aware she was going in for an operation and I remember going into the local pub with Chris. People kept coming up to him saying they could not believe what she was doing and he had to sit down and explain it all to me. It was never made into a big deal, more a case that she had to go into hospital to make sure she was going to be all right in the future. It was never over-dramatised because in her own words she could never do that.'

'I told her I did not want to die', Wendy recalled in a very matter of fact way. 'I told her I didn't want to end up like some

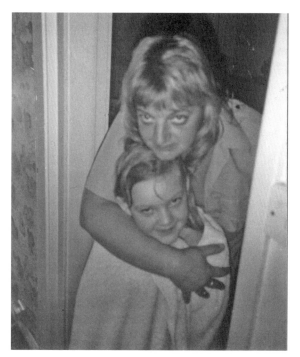

Becky at five years old with her Mum

of the other relatives and this operation would stop that happening. That was the only way I could tell her what was going on; the truth is always the simplest way. She knew exactly what I was having done. She was made aware there was nothing to worry about and there was no big fuss to be made.'

It was an approach Becky appreciated at the time. The news had spread to the rest of the village and people were asking questions, but she knew what was happening and did not need protecting from that. The way Wendy dealt with it was to allow her the opportunity of dealing with it herself. Becky picked up the baton and ran with it

'Mum had to be pragmatic about it to be able to get to that stage in the first place. She would not have got anywhere by getting all hysterical. I remember more about other people's reactions, a sense of shock and asking if she was OK.

I remember telling them all she was fine and I was going to see her tonight; probably appearing very blasé about the whole thing. What I remember most was that I wanted a pair of Doc Marten shoes but mum never let me have them. When she went into hospital Chris treated me to a pair and I remember going to see her in hospital and she just said to me, ''What are those on your feet?'' I remember her crying on one occasion because she was happy. She was sat in a room full of people waiting to be diagnosed with cancer, wondering how long they had got to live and all she had to wait for was a lift home.'

Becky dealt with it head on, an attitude she would need to replicate. The implication of the genetic research had severe repercussions for Becky which she may not have considered. Not many teenagers have to reflect on the possibility of developing of a killer disease; this was the question that would be put to her.

'Around the time of my mum having the operation, I was unaware of any risk to myself. I remember knowing about it later when she first did her publicity, but it was well explained to me. I used to talk to people at school when I was 14 because they would come and ask me about it. I told them I had a 50 per cent chance of having breast cancer and would reel off these percentages to them. At the time it was so normal for me but looking back it must be a strange thing to come out with for a child. I'm surprised they didn't turn it into some sort of maths lesson.'

This familiarity with one of the UK's biggest killers allowed her to make sense of what had happened. Wendy's attitude rubbed off on Becky, giving her the freedom to discuss it with her friends as if it were an after-school topic and banish any concerns about her mother's health. The operation was over and was not something that Becky had to confront for some time. However, Becky would have to deal with more questions and more facts as her mother went public with her experiences. A future radio presenter was about to get her first taste of media exposure.

The *Independent* article opened up a new world for Wendy, one that Becky was very much a part of it. By this time the gene theory was developing and many of the journalists, photographers and radio interviewers were keen to get Becky involved as part of Wendy's story. It was another adventure for a teenager who had already experienced more than most people do in a lifetime.

'I think it was more the fact that mum was famous. I was 13 years old and mum was in the papers. The phones went ballistic and I wasn't allowed to answer them, but one day she told me she had got a call from *The Big Breakfast* on Channel 4 and that was it for me. I told her she had to go and it was probably pressure from me that made her do that particular show because I wanted to go with her. It probably never dawned on me that all this was because of breast cancer; it was more just being able to boast to my friends and watch my mum on telly. As a teenager it does not get any better than that.'

Becky had been turned into a celebrity in her own school. It exposed her to a new world but the reality was that not a great deal had changed. She was used to being questioned about her mother due to the local reaction to her operation and enjoyed being in the limelight. As every teenager faces a battle to be noticed in the crowd, Becky revelled in the attention it gave her. It gave her the edge at a vital age, while everybody else was talking about which boy they fancied or which film star they wanted to snog, Becky was going on *The Big Breakfast* with her mum.

The publicity did not win favour with everyone. Becky's father, Jeremy, had serious reservations about how this would affect their daughter at what he believed was an important stage of her life. It certainly was not down to ignorance; his mother suffered badly from the disease and also suffered ovarian cancer before dying of throat cancer. He knew all about how this terrible sickness can tear apart a family. After splitting from Wendy in 1988 he knew all about her fierce attitude to breast cancer and how she would do all she could to try and prevent others suffering like her mother. Jeremy understood the purpose of going public with her experiences; he did not see why it had to involve Becky.

'My concerns were that Becky was being pushed into this at too early an age because she was always with Wendy

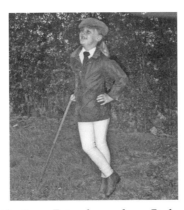

Unafraid – Long Eaton horse show; Becky at seven

throughout the publicity. Whether it was on television or in the paper, people used to come up to me and say they had seen my daughter on telly again. I was worried rather than annoyed and between the ages of 11 and 15 my feelings were mixed because Becky had not been diagnosed at that stage. I am and always have been a keen supporter of breast cancer research, I saw my mother go through absolute agony before she died so I know what it can do. I just thought it was a bit early for Becky. I thought she was too young.'

Wendy disagrees and believes she was right to continue to allow her daughter full involvement in what was happening.

'When anybody asked if they could speak to Becky or take a photograph I said yes. She was well into double figures when we discovered the family history and the publicity did not come out until two years after I had the operation. I thought there was nothing for her to worry about and she was about 13 years old when the publicity first began to take off. She was old enough to be talking about things and it was never something we kept a secret. I never made a big fuss about it, therefore there was never anything to hide.'

Becky was caught in the middle. Like many teenagers both parents were looking out for her and had different ideas on how to approach the situation. Jeremy had never been comfortable with the media and there was always talk about new miracle cures that were being tested and could be available in the future.

It was difficult for him to watch his little girl with the thought that she may be heading for the same operation one day. But a youngster who was hungry for attention and wanted to be involved in her fight for awareness could not accept the caution he displayed.

'It was difficult because I could see where he was coming from but in another respect I was living a different life from the one I had when I went to see him. As a young girl you do not want to talk to your dad about your boobs, whether it was in the papers or not it is embarrassing. It's not that I wanted him phased out of the experience, there are just some things that are easier to talk about with your mum.

'I fought to get into those pictures. There was no suggestion that my mum used me to further her cause because it was not needed. Helen could have been involved, she was the same generation as me and I remember being mortified when mum took her to go on "Anne and Nick". I was distraught that she went there without me. My mum could see the benefit in being involved with the media because it wasn't a taboo subject and it was never kept quiet between us. We were being open and that was how she wanted it to be. If anything it made me confident in my ability to talk about it and certainly helped me in the future.'

Wendy was becoming heavily involved in raising awareness. She was very busy with her various appearances on TV and radio, not to mention her increasing involvement with the family planning clinic. Once again the perception of a normal right of passage from childhood to adulthood was not there for Becky as outside influences took her mother's attention away. Their dual involvement in the publicity helped to bridge that gap and kept them together more than if Becky had elected to take a back seat. She admits that nothing was ever what your average child would call normal.

'My mum brought out a single, she ran a shop, set up a theatre company, became involved in showjumping and I was part of all those things. I don't think it was ever a case of not getting her attention because I was quite good at being able to stamp my feet and do that. She was extremely busy in most aspects, especially in terms of setting up the helpline. People would come round to the house all the time, but I enjoyed being in close proximity to people I had not met before. It was like meeting the new family members all over again. I never felt exploited and my mum liked me to be involved in all the exposure because I was involved in what she was doing. It was good fun, very fast moving, but there was nothing wrong with that. It's how I like it.'

Becky knew only too well by then that one day she would have a decision to make. Watching her mother choose to go through surgery to avoid breast cancer had proved to her just what a vile disease this was. The way she came out of the operation with such energy and vigour to raise awareness gave her the perception that the procedure did not even come close to matching the severity of the consequences of not taking it on. Wendy had cleared the way for others to follow in her footsteps and Becky had been with her on her journey. It was never going to be an easy ride but it allowed her to move through her teenage years with her eyes wide open to the choices she may have to face.

'Mum has pioneered what she fought for and been a focus for a lot of people and I am extremely honoured to have someone like that as my mum, not that I would ever tell her that. I would never have had the strength to push like she has. If someone had told me what the GPs told her, I would have just accepted it. I grew up knowing that breast cancer could lay in wait. There was no feeling that it was suddenly sprung on me at the age of 19. I felt I could handle anything and I will always be very grateful that mum kept me informed all the way. There was no big sit down chat. It sounds like an old film cliché, but I was told on a need-to-know basis and it prepared me for what was to come.'

The focus of media attention was changing. Becky was approaching the age of consent for the gene test and there was a huge interest in what would happen. Wendy had been in control of all the information that was being put out through the newspapers. Her experience with *Bella* had convinced her that not all outlets were as desperate as she was in the cause to raise awareness. This was the one thing that Becky had no experience or concept of. Jeremy's concern that she could succumb to the

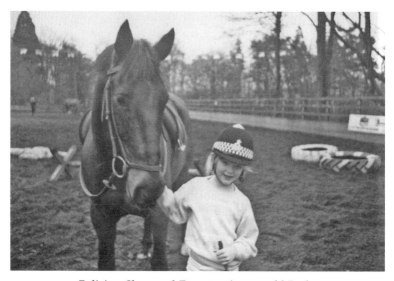

Policing Sherwood Forest – six year old Becky

evils of press attention would be realised in a *Sunday People* article, just as she passed her 17th birthday.

'The headline was "I'm 17 and I Want My Breasts Removed", which was not the case at all. My belief was that I would have the genetic test in time, maybe leave it past my 18th birthday and if a cure had not been found, then I will have the operation. They did not portray it that way at all. I was in the sixth form at school and it had an impact because a lot of people believe what they read in the papers and looked at me differently. The good thing was I got to go on "GMTV" the next morning and put the record straight.'

'Mum always told me to tell the truth and be honest. She was keen to keep it uplifting and not to turn it into a negative. Whenever pictures were taken they would always try and get you to pull the sad face and mum would be a nightmare. She would smile to prove a point. I did get over-cautious because they would press points that were not important, things about my love life. I was very naïve about it and it was very humiliating. The story was OK but the sensational headline with a double spread and a picture of me took it all out of context, saying I was following in my mother's footsteps. I learnt the hard way but it just made me more determined to put the record straight.'

Becky had made close friends who knew what was happening. Approaching 18 she did all the things most teenagers do when they approach adulthood and begin socialising. It was also when she began her first serious relationship. She had been best friends with Hayley Price since she started at Lady Manners School in Bakewell at the age of 11 and she had already had a first kiss with her brother Carl when she was 12 at the back of a bus. They began mixing in the same circle and things became a little more serious. A relationship was beginning to form that would see her through some of her darkest days.

'I had known him since I was young and we got together after my 18th birthday. It was all very awkward because I had to admit to Hayley that I thought her brother was quite good looking; very embarrassing because her reaction was just to shout "No way". We saw each other for a bit and it was in the March after my birthday when we got together. He played hard to get for a while before I got my claws into him. We hung around with the same group of eight or so friends and we were the ones that got together.'

For Becky it was an ideal coupling. She describes Carl as a very sensible and organised person; loves a good night out with his friends and is the opposite of Becky in many ways. By his own admission he likes to stay out of the limelight and offers Becky a firm grounding by way of emotional support and stopping her from getting carried away with the publicity. Because of how Becky and Hayley used to talk, Carl knew all about how breast cancer could affect his other half in the very near future. He was under no illusions.

'I knew most of the basics through my sister anyway but I did not know much about it from a detailed point of view. When we started hanging around together we used to talk about it a bit and it went from there. She explained more as time went on. It was actually when she started talking about taking the gene test and asked me whether I thought she should have it and how old she should be, that the talks became more serious.

We just talked about it from there really. There was never anything massive to talk about because nothing was really happening before then.'

'At the time we got together', Becky recalls, 'it was not a big issue and the gene test was not available to me before I was 18 anyway. I thought it was going to be way, way in the future but it was never something we discussed or I thought he was worried about. I don't think his opinion has changed much in that time anyway. He would tell me that I needed to get it sorted and I would say that I knew. The way we talked things through was similar to how my mum dealt with me, very gradual. What Carl did well was to comfort me if I came back after a night out and asked him if he thought having the test was a good idea. We were a good double act.'

When to have the all-important gene test was not addressed in Becky's teenage years. Instead she decided to get her career sorted out and, fresh from her brush with the media world that filled her so full of excitement, became a promotions girl at Peak FM, a radio station in Chesterfield. She started in May and by October had impressed enough to be offered an on-air position as co-host of the breakfast show, the station's flagship programme. Her early exposure to the media world had earned its second positive goal. As well as helping her deal with the problems she was soon to face, she had crossed to the other side of the broadcasting line.

'Rob Birnie was the breakfast presenter at the time and it was Wayne Chadwick who gave me my big break. Rob left before too long and Sean Goldsmith took over in January after I had been there for just four months. We were a little wary of each other to start with. It was harder for Sean because he had been in the business for a long time and was working with someone who only had a few months experience and was still making the obvious mistakes. We have got on very well since then and created a good on-air chemistry that we call the brother and sister relationship. We can have ago at each other because we love each other really.'

'Initially it was quite hard', recalls Sean about the first few months of working with Becky on the breakfast show. 'She was new into the job and I expected too much from her from the word go. I am an impatient person so it was quite tough for me to assume she would be at the level that I expected, but after a couple of months it just clicked. It came together overnight and she has grown into the role as a person as well as a presenter.'

It was a defining move in dealing with her predicament. Becky was on the way to becoming a key figure in the fight to change the direction of cancer research, although to start with her new career masked the situation in hand. The gene test was still waiting to be carried out, even though it had been available to her for the past two years. She had talked it through with Carl, Wendy and Jeremy, who were all anxious for her to go through with it sooner rather than later. It was not until she was 22 that the comfort barrier came crashing down when she found out her cousin Helen had developed breast cancer at just 29 years of age.

'I was interviewed on GMTV about the genetic testing just three months before Helen was diagnosed. They asked if I would consider having the test, bearing in mind my mum already knew she carried the gene. I said that I was thinking about taking it in a few years time but that there was no rush. I wanted to sort out my life insurance and also live a little because, as far as I was concerned, it was a decision that was still some way off, probably towards my late twenties, which was still seven or eight years away. I was also conscious that there were all sorts of medical advances that could be made by then. I did not take it as seriously as I should have done. What happened to Helen changed all that. Doing nothing was no longer an option.'

The risk of breast cancer was thrust forwards in devastating fashion. It was no longer a matter for discussion. Despite the simplicity of the procedure, no more complicated than a blood test, the implications of what it can reveal are serious. At Becky's age, you cannot just decide to take the test because of what is at stake, there is a lot more to think about, not least your own mental preparation An appointment had to be made at St Mary's Hospital in Manchester where Professor Gareth Evans was to become again something other than a family friend and re-take his position as medical expert.

'First of all, is it the right option for you at that particular time? The test will be there in the future. Do you want to know whether you have a high risk in your lifetime as early as your twenties, because you might not be prepared to do anything about it? You cannot go for early screening because mammograms do not work properly under the age of 30, so a very difficult decision could be forced on you. Are you ready to face what is a very high risk? Also, there are issues such as

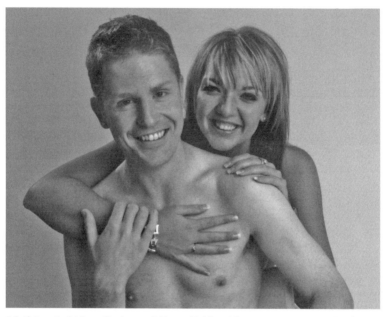

Nothing to hide – Becky and Sean Goldsmith, co-presenters at Peak FM

insurance. At the moment insurance companies are not allowed to use these tests for calculating premiums, but they often find ways of finding out about your family history. If they discover you are at risk of a potentially deadly disease they could penalise you, so you need to sort your insurance out before taking the test. What are you going to do with this information? Are you going to consider early surgery? Obviously, in Becky's case, this was the main reason for considering the test. She probably would not have gone ahead with the test unless she had an option like surgery to deal with it, because she felt she could then embark on something she knew was going to make a very substantial difference to that risk. Wendy had paved the way for people to take this up rather than just sit there and worry about it. Becky felt this was a reason for her to go ahead with the test. She had a very definite choice she could make with the results.'

Becky was in the perfect position to further raise awareness of the genetic issue. Presenters and staff at Peak FM were familiar with the fact that she might discover that the family gene could put her at risk of developing breast cancer. In her time there she had become a much-loved personality and had built up a strong fan base of listeners, partly because she was the only female voice on the station and had the ability to relate to the listeners with her local roots. It was clear to everyone within the station that she would face her own personal drama. In a media world where drama sells newspapers and builds up an audience, it could prove beneficial to play this out over the airwaves. In light of what Wendy had done to raise awareness, it also represented an opportunity for Becky to go public and continue her efforts to make people understand what breast cancer can do.

'I did not see the benefit of keeping it quiet and there was a public interest, much like there had been with mum and she has helped so many people. The publicity was something I had grown up with and never thought anything of, until I was put in a similar situation and could look back and realise what an incredible woman she is and what she had accomplished. I saw the good it did her and thought that keeping my situation quiet would be no good for anybody. It was time to repay my mother's good work by carrying it on. On top of all that it would make damn good radio, help The Genesis Appeal, and Sean felt the same.

'It was something we talked about off air', Sean agreed, 'and the way radio works you try to put your own life across without giving too much detail away. It just seemed like a brilliant story and we knew she was going to take the test so we followed it knowing the audience would follow it with us. Becky did not want to shy away from it and it helped everything from the profile of The Genesis Appeal to Becky herself.'

It wasn't just Peak FM who wanted to take the story on. The *Tonight With Trevor MacDonald* crew had filmed Helen through her operation and Siobhan Sinnerton, who was the producer of the show, had became aware of the genetic theories coming out of St Mary's Hospital from Professor Evans. They were interested in following somebody through the process of getting a positive gene test, deciding on the next course of action and taking it through to its conclusion. Having already followed one young woman through a test that resulted in her getting the all clear, her attention was drawn to Becky.

'I did the initial programme about breast cancer two years before Becky's genetic test and we looked at a variety of different case studies. One of those was her cousin Helen who we followed through her experiences along with the whole family history issue. It was then that I became aware of the gene-testing programme in Manchester, which I thought would make a fascinating piece. We approached staff at St Mary's and spoke to Genesis saying we would like to follow someone through the whole process and they eventually put us onto Becky. I had met her once before when we were filming Helen on one of the occasions that she went for her radiotherapy treatment.

'The issue of gene testing seemed like an incredibly interesting subject and I wanted to portray the science behind it and the advances that were being made in a very human way. It struck me that she was only 23 years old and had an incredible journey to take with some phenomenal choices for someone who was so young. On top of that, once I knew from meeting her that she had such an amazing personality I knew there was the making of a really good film there.'

The scene appeared to be set. The choice seemed to have been made and the appointment was booked to have the gene test in January 2004. There was no question of waiting to see if the gene would catch up with her the way it caught up with Helen. A real-life drama was to be played out over the radio airwaves and the nation's TV screens; there would be no possible way of avoiding the issue. It was time to find out if there was a decision to make and what the outcome of that decision would be.

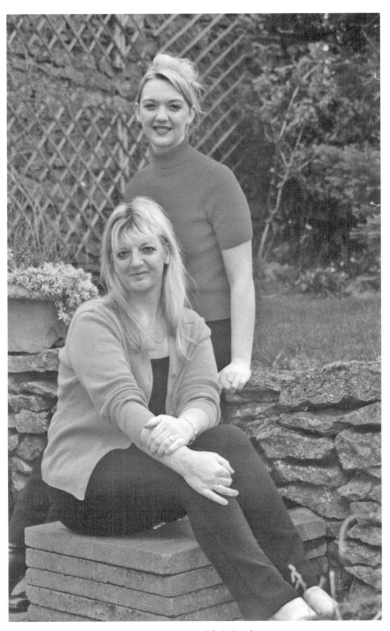

Becky at 17 with Wendy

NO BIG DEAL

'There wasn't much to fear from the genetic test, but there was one thing that kept going through my head in the few days before taking it. I had planned for everything and thought I was prepared but then it suddenly hit me. What would I do if it came back negative?'

Most people would be delighted by that outcome. Becky was convinced she had an 80 to 85 per cent of getting breast cancer, to have that weight lifted and remove the need for a preventive operation would surely be the best case scenario. However, Becky was not most people and had spent the last five or six years with her mindset geared towards having to deal with a positive test. It was a belief she was having difficulty unplugging from and to be faced with the knowledge that there was still a one in ten risk of getting breast cancer without the gene may have proved harder to accept. Being faced with the prospect of not having the gene threw up other doubts.

'Would I be OK about it, thinking I was going to get something for a good part of my life and then suddenly having that taken away from me? I wondered if I might feel a bit lost and wondered if I would be even more paranoid about the whole breast cancer thing and about my health if the gene was not there. It was even in my thoughts on the way to the hospital when I discussed it with my mum and she told me that if I didn't want the results, I did not have to have them and could think about other alternatives.'

Becky would never consider changing her mind. The shock of finding out her cousin Helen had been diagnosed at 29 made sure of that and the test was taken in January 2004. After spending her whole adult life with breast cancer lurking in the shadows, Becky finally had time to think about what was happening in the few weeks between taking the test and finding out the result. Niggling doubts began creeping in and a level of uncertainty into how thing may pan out. Suddenly the realisation that the future might not be mapped out in the way they had all suspected was all too real. However, the doubts did not extend to the actual taking of the test.

'I had told everybody, all the listeners as well. There were plenty of family members to relate to and the theory was that the genetic test was the start of things for me, not the end. At the very worst it was just being told that I had a faulty gene and that never frightened me. It was not something I had to sit at home and worry about and was nothing compared to the operation. There was never any question of me changing my mind; I was just too impatient. I had my blood taken and I wanted to find out the next day. If I could have found out in the next hour I would have been more than happy.'

At 22, Becky would discover how her future would be mapped out. Would the results lead to life changing surgery or just a population risk of breast cancer? In her mind it was difficult to reason which outcome would be the better of the two, but her reaction to the results surprised everyone.

'I laughed. I had tears coming out of my eyes but I was laughing. The feeling was like having this sudden urge to giggle at the most inappropriate moment but you cannot help it. I was being told that something as serious as breast cancer would more than likely feature in my near future and all I could do was giggle. I think I was fine with the results and just wanted to move on. The laughter was more relief. I felt this huge deep breath come from inside me, felt my shoulders sag to the point where I was a bit light headed because after all these years I finally knew. This was something I had spoken about time and time again and to finally know was a peculiar feeling.'

Becky was not alone in dealing with the situation. Relatives wanted to know, lots of friends, workmates and listeners, not to mention staff that were there to break the news, many of whom had become family friends. Becky took it better than most.

'Mum was upset but there was nothing she could do about it, it had never crossed my mind that it was anybody's fault. Gareth Evans, who broke the news to me was upset, as he would be, he has been a family friend since I was 11 and it must have been a difficult thing to pass on. Some of my friends did not take it too brilliantly, the majority were fine but the odd one had a few tears, although I told a lot of them by text message. My half sister was quite upset and my dad was concerned with what I would do next because he had not lived with it the way I had. Helen was Helen, just upset because she would rather I didn't have it but she told me that she knew I would cope more than anyone.'

The ITV1 crew captured the scene. They were hoping to follow Becky through the entire process and for producer Siobhan Sinnerton there was mixed feelings about someone she was only just beginning to get to know. After two previous cases had tested negative, Becky provided them with the opportunity to proceed with the filming. But there was also the integrity of the moment to consider.

'She expected it would be positive until those doubts at the end. I had no idea what to expect. It was quite upsetting because she was faced with such incredible odds of getting breast cancer at such a young age. It was not a very nice place to be, to be in the room with someone who was getting news like that, but ironically it meant that we would go on this journey together. It is hard for people who don't know the detailed knowledge of people with hereditary breast cancer to understand, but there was a kind of relief about getting that positive result because if she had a negative one, she would never have seen these doctors again which disturbed her as well. At least this way she could make the decision to eradicate the threat and deal with it her way.'

'I knew that if I had the gene', Becky recollected, 'then I would have the operation. I had seen my mum go through it, seen others have it done and watched them recover, so I knew there was a strong network of people around me, stronger than most families, and I knew it was what I was going to do. I wanted to make sure for my own piece of mind that I had considered all the options and looked at everything, just so I could have that comfort and I did delve into it and research it fully.

'I always tried to look on the brighter side as soon as I got the results and joked about having the opportunity to have a perfect pair of boobs. The breast nurse, who told me in no uncertain terms that this was definitely not a boob job, very quickly told me off. I knew it wasn't, it was just my way of speaking about it and making light of the situation, but that was all part of the counselling.'

Becky decided not to rush into setting a date. A mastectomy and reconstruction was not a process to take lightly and having waited this long to find out the news, she continued to research the options. Time was a factor but Professor Evans praised Becky for her thoroughness.

'We certainly do not want people rushing into a decision like surgery. It is a huge choice to make and they have to be absolutely and properly prepared for it. We find that when women have done that, had a proper psychological assessment, seen the surgeon and planned things out, under those circumstances they are much better equipped to go through the process. I think it is essential that women do take time thinking about it, knowing what the potential problems could be.'

Becky soon decided on the specific course of action. Her mother had a complete mastectomy and has yet to go through reconstruction, but for all their similarities, Becky had a different plan of attack. After much deliberation she opted for a procedure referred to as a 'Bi-lateral Preventative Mastectomy with Reconstruction and Preservation of the Nipples'. This would involve removing as much of the breast tissue as possible, have a level of reconstructive surgery at the same time, leaving the nipple on the end of a vascular stalk so that it can be preserved above the implants. What this would essentially mean is that a risk of breast cancer would still remain.

'I chose to have the reconstruction as well because of my age. Image is a factor for me and I knew how surgery had progressed. It was possible to do it and I knew the risk would be minimal, reduced to about 8 per cent, still below the population risk. Retaining the nipples as well was something I wanted to do to keep just that little bit of me. If in the future I did not want them anymore then I could go and have them removed at a later date. I felt more comfortable with it, which was the most important thing, and I would be checked every year for the rest of my life.'

Becky went public with her decision in June 2004. She got back from a holiday with friends in Zante in Greece and went on the BBC TV's 'East Midlands Today' programme, which did a piece about her plans for the operation. Her life would never be the same again. Calls came flooding in from newspapers ranging from the *Derbyshire Times* to the *Daily Mail*. National radio stations got in touch; ITN, fivenews and Sky News were also interested. There was attention from overseas with organisations from Spain and the United States ringing her up. The media circus had come to town. The reaction from the listeners on Peak FM was also phenomenal and for a short while the tide was in danger of engulfing Becky as everybody wanted to know why she was having an operation to remove her breasts when she was not ill. Everywhere she turned there was a reaction.

'All these people that I don't even know, some didn't even listen to the station, but the response was absolutely amazing. To be told that I was helping other people as well from the e-mails and phone calls was the most amazing feeling. I was being called an inspiration and you cannot get any better than that. I had e-mails from people I had and hadn't met who told me they were behind me 100 per cent. OK, there were some people who were not helpful and didn't think I was doing the right thing; that I was rushing into it. I have always said this operation is not right for everyone, but it was right for me, it was my right choice.'

The decision angered some people. Some of the e-mails told her to stop eating meat, drink more fruit juice or turn to God. A small proportion of people reacted in a way that was almost accusatory and used her situation to champion their own cause, be it moral or religious. It was something that Becky was not prepared to shy away from and such reactions were confronted in the manner in which they were sent.

'I want to carry on with my life and just be normal like everyone else and I believed that having this operation would give me that option. Every person who wrote in, I gave them time but I had made my mind up. Fair enough, if that was what people want to do and that was what they believed in, who am I to stand in their way? But by the same extension this was my choice. It was only a couple of people who actually got cross because I didn't choose their way. It was a bit out of order, these people trying to tell me that what they had done was right and nothing else counted. Fair enough, they believed what they did, but do not push it on other people.'

There was also cynicism directed towards her choice. Coming from a media background the accusations that Becky was going through with this to further her career were uttered. There were also those who said she was only going through with it because her mother had it done. This was always greeted with consternation from Becky who regarded such accusations with contempt.

'Some did say it was a publicity stunt, never to my face of course, but who goes and has major surgery of this type just to get attention? I did not even know what the end result was going to be like. I did get one lady who asked what my boyfriend thought about what I was having done. I told her he was fine and loved me. She told me that her husband said that if she ever had anything like that done then he would leave her. I asked her if that meant he would rather have you six feet under than alive without a pair of boobs and she said "yes". I was gobsmacked, but you have to hold your tongue because it is not my place to tell people how they should live their lives.'

It was a side of going public that was not entirely unexpected. When Wendy became involved with the media there were people who wanted to pour scorn on her decision, this was a similar scenario that brought similar criticisms. Fortunately for Becky she had developed a thick skin and a strong network of friends who helped her through the more difficult moments. There was a sense of people wanting to get to know Becky because of who she was, others believing that by becoming friendly with Becky they could get free CDs from the radio stations, become involved in TV interviews and satisfy their own egos. Becky's social circle closed ranks and made sure things did not get out of hand on a night out or social engagement. Nicky Bacon, who lives in Bakewell has been friends with Becky since she was 14 and she remembers one particular occasion.

'There was a stage before the operation, during one of the calendar launches in Brampton, when there were some nasty comments from two elderly women because they thought

Becky had not dealt with breast cancer and was able to prevent it. They must have gone through it and maybe felt bitter about the attention she was getting. Some people do not understand it and think it's been easy for her. It is frustrating when you hear people talk about her like that because as her friends we know what she has gone through; being with her when she found out she had the gene right through to the operation. I did feel we had to protect her from people who might upset her and that was a perfect case in point. She does not want confrontation and never retaliated, she just accepts that some people simply do not understand and tries to ignore it.'

The preparation for the operation would be as much mental as physical. There was a lot of counselling and much to consider because, although Becky new all about the disease and its consequences, the operation was a different matter. She would have to understand that she was about to lose a part of her body she would never get back. Becky visited psychiatrists, counsellors, her surgeon Andy Baildam and breast nurse Lesley Thompson several times to make sure she understood what would be involved in the process and what risks the operation would pose. It was Lesley who laid it on the line for Becky and gave her the bare facts about what she was about to put herself through.

'A big role for me at St Mary's is to play devil's advocate. I feel like a horrible person at times because I have to give them the nitty-gritty, which is that the word 'reconstruction' means her breasts will be false. It is easy for women to kid themselves that they have had their breasts cut off but will not really lose them because when they wake up it will be as if nothing has happened. It is not at all like that, you will be changed, you will be different and things will never be the same again. My only fear was that she was so up-front and so sure of what she was doing that I wondered if she would get a feeling of anti-climax at the end. I was worried she would be let down and actually find herself mourning her breasts; something she may not have thought about but I have seen it happen.'

Becky was made aware of worse case scenarios and asked difficult questions. She was asked how she would feel if they could not save her nipples during the operation or if she would end up with nothing. She was made aware that she would not be able to breast feed her future children. There were mammograms that needed to be performed, psychological assessments that needed to be carried out. She had to be made aware that there was a recovery period and further operations likely, due to the nature of the reconstruction. It was not an easy period but a date had been set with her surgeon Andy Baildam. The operation was booked in June 2005, just over a year after going public with the decision to take preventive surgery. The build up began in earnest on that day and there was a long time to wait until 26 January 2006.

'Mentally I knew I was doing the right thing by having the operation and I could rationalise it perfectly. From an emotional viewpoint I found that long build up to the operation very difficult. Mum and Helen had both told me how they felt this huge sense of relief afterwards, but for me it was very different. I did not have breast cancer as Helen did and had not

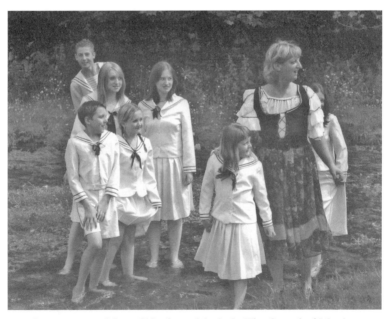

A courageous Mum: Wendy as Maria in The Sound of Music –
High Peak Performance at Buxton Opera House in 2004

experienced anyone dying of it in the way my mum had. It was not that I thought I was making the wrong decision, but I had such a long time to dwell on it and I just wanted it done.'

Part of the concern was how she would look afterwards. Becky has a very strong sense of her self-image and despite her willingness to have both breasts removed, it would be wrong to think she did not care about the after effects. Whereas Wendy had a perception of her breasts as inviting cancer to strike and confessed to having no pleasure in that part of her body, Becky's view was very different. As a young woman in a physical relationship it was important to at least have some idea of what she would look like after the operation. Shortly after setting a date for the big day, Becky and Carl paid another visit to Lesley Thompson at the Withington Hospital in Manchester. She was able to put them in the picture as to what might lie in store for her.

'I was concerned about what Carl might think because I had seen mastectomies before, the good and the bad ones, but Carl had never seen one. I found that a bit hard at first until I went to see Lesley who showed us pictures of the outcome and he said they looked really good. For me that was it. I just told them to get on with the operation because I knew that Carl was 100 per cent behind me and that we would come out of it the other side none the worse for the experience. He has always been a total support, it never crossed my mind for one minute that he would leave me if things did go wrong because I know that men are fantastic. We do not give them enough credit.'

'Seeing the photos did get me a bit at first', Carl admits. 'We did not actually see any photos properly of people who had been through the same operation as Becky, it was more along the lines of people who had cancer and that was a slightly different procedure. That did set me up for expecting the worst of what could happen and then we saw the shots of a girl who had reconstruction and it was two years down the line. All the scarring had gone down and they looked fantastic and that brought your hopes up that the results could be absolutely amazing. It was interesting and we were glad we saw them before she went under the knife because it brought it home what could potentially happen to her.'

Lesley recalled the meeting and how it was a turning point in Becky's mindset. By knowing that Carl was excited about the outcome it put many of her own fears to the back of her mind and that was half of the battle. The visual impact of what would happen to her was no longer an unknown. Lesley is well aware it can go either way.

'It is a lot to face up to for people, but every woman experiences it in a different way. Becky was relatively detached at the time, but being shown the photographs is often the point where an awful lot of women get tearful and worried. The pictures often make them remember their mothers, and in many cases it was breast cancer that had killed them, which was not the case in Becky's situation. It was a great step forward in a sense but a lot of women in Becky's position will have gone through their teenage years with a loved one having had very mutilating surgery and getting more and more ill. You see a great outpouring of emotion. Becky was less emotional about that, almost intellectually interested in the workings; figuring out the process itself rather than treating it as something that would happen to her.'

Becky tried to live her life as normally as possible, but in the six months leading up to the operation this proved to be a bit more difficult. She began treating everything as a landmark and began experimenting with her own femininity, including hair extensions. There was a sense that, for a short time at least, the knowledge that part of her body was about to be lost may have started to catch up with her. There was also the documentary crew who continued filming in between the gene test and operation. The programme was not just about focusing on the scientific and medical side but also to get a sense of how the decision making process affected her emotionally. It was something that Wendy initially had a few concerns about.

'There was such a lot of media about her, with the radio station and ITV. There was always a sense that this was the last this, this was the last that, the last night out, last holiday, last day at work. I was not sure all that was such a good idea. It was starting to make a really big event of the operation and that had never been the case for me, I just made a decision and got on with it. This was being built into a drama and it had been never promoted in that way, in fact we went out of our way to down play it. I was not convinced this was the best way forward.'

'We had to look at the landmarks of her decision making process', explained Siobhan Sinnerton, the ITV producer. 'I also wanted to get a sense of her as a person, her work life, social life, her relationship with the audience and how they were such a part of this. I understand people's concerns because having a camera is an intrusion in itself but there was never any awkwardness. There were times when I chose to turn the camera off and let her do things in private, like when she got the results of the test for example. We followed her home and had her telling other people, but I did not know her well enough doing that and she needed some private time.'

All was well until a month before the operation. It was New Year's Eve when the jitters really set in and once again it was psychological rather than fear of the operation. After months of going through the preparation, Becky could no longer refer to the operation as something that would take place next year. The realisation that it was only a few weeks away became a little too much.

'Some people hate New Year because it reminds them of some of the bad things that have happened in the previous 12 months. I have never looked at things that way, I prefer to look forward and that was why when we heard Big Ben strike 12 it just hit me. The operation had seemed so far away before, now it was almost here and I had my friends and Carl with me, had a little too much to drink and I started crying about it. I was looking forward to something that was going to change my life in the same way other people get upset about looking back and I realised I needed the support of everyone who was there that night. When the DJ played *That's What Friends Are For* by Dionne Warwick it set us all off, it must have looked so strange for anyone not in my groups of friends watching a big group of girls crying their eyes out on New Year's Day.'

It was all starting to get a little bit too real. Becky became concerned that her friends were getting fed up hearing about the operation. Fears about the procedure began to swamp her but she bottled it up in front of her friends. There was still no question of her going through with the surgery but she needed reassurance. Her mother had spent her whole life trying to make light of the situation, playing it down so that Becky would not become concerned. It was time for a serious chat.

'I did keep teasing Becky in a way because at one stage it was probably the way to do it, but then she became more tense. One day she came in and told me she was scared and sobbed in front of me. That was very, very hard and at that point I was probably like any mum would be. I told her it would all be alright, told her she did not need to go for the operation now and it was hard for me to see her like that a month before. She started to read the Caron Keating book, read the first chapter and then said she knew it was the right decision. She came to it by herself, the little indecision she had she just suddenly overcame it and then became very calm.'

Messages of support from listeners came as a great comfort. Many of them recalled their own experiences of cancer, many of them in a positive way. The e-mails, texts and cards allowed her to realise that she was not alone in going through with this operation.

'I had loads of e-mails from people locally who had similar experiences, operations or even breast cancer themselves. So many women said I was doing the right thing and were supportive. It was lovely because I had mails from people who talked me through the operation and told me what they had done. Some explained that it might feel a little strange at first but not to worry because I would get used to it and everything would become normal. It was so lovely to be able to talk to people I did not know so openly and it really helped in the weeks leading up to the operation. I was not about to let any of them down.'

Those e-mails were as much an inspiration to Becky as they claimed she was to them. Here is a selection of some that were sent just before the operation.

Some times we think we really know some people, but we don't know really know them at all ... but the funny thing is that we all had a baby last year for Sean [Becky's co-presenter] ... we all went into labour for his wife ... and now we are all praying for strength for Becky.... What an inspiration to all young ladies having the same op or facing it.

Karen, Old Whittington

Hope your operation goes well Becky, we will all be thinking about you. Keep your chin up darling. Sean, I am sure you'll be lost without her so Becky hurry back cause you make a great twosome.

Louise, Staveley

Good luck Becks from everyone here at Sheepbridge Cricket Club. By the way, does this mean that your page on next year's calendar will be supersized!!!

Wavey, Sheepbridge.

Thank you very much Becky. My mum and my sister both died of breast cancer, I'm now going for my gene test. I was too scared before but you really are a life saver because I'm going because of you.

What Becky was doing provoked a response in everybody. Her life over the past two years had been played out on Peak FM and there were many thousands of people who were going through with it with her. As a consequence the realities hit home for many people, including her co-presenter Sean, on her last day. The ITV1 crew were there for what would prove to be a surprisingly emotional day.

'When you are a man you try and keep emotions intact but as the time approached 10 o'clock, just before the news, I had a little speech prepared. I was going to say something like "You are Becky Measures. You are my little sister." Something like that. I just could not get the words out, I got about three words in and Becky, whose voice was already cracking up, just said "Don't do it Goldsmith, just don't do it." There was a bit of a pause and I just went to the news, there was nothing I could say to sum it up. I know the camera crew were filling up as well; it was a very emotional morning. I was not expecting that because it never really hit home before that day; it was just Becky.'

The countdown was almost complete. Becky had said her goodbyes to her workmates, organised a big send-off to her friends and relatives the previous weekend in Chesterfield. She had even gone through her wardrobe and said a few ceremonial goodbyes to some of the outfits that may not suit what would be a newly shaped Becky. All that was left to do now was go to the hospital and check in.

It was about two o'clock on Wednesday 25 January that she set foot in The Nightingale Centre in Manchester for the first time as a patient. Her room was very bare and clinical, not at all homely, a detail that did little to take her mind off what would happen to her the very next day. Before any formal talk of anaesthetic and surgical procedures could take place, a personalisation of the room was in order as Carl and Wendy put up cards. Breast cancer would be a thing of the past before it had a chance to be a part of her present, a fact that contributed to a growing sense of surrealism about the experience.

'It did not feel real at all, going into hospital when I wasn't ill or hurt but knew that I was going to be; that was odd. It was kind of like knowing you are going to break your leg and it is going to damn well hurt. I didn't like that but it was all part of how things felt in those few weeks leading up to that moment. You always hear people say you do not know how people feel about a person until they die. I've kind of had that experience but whilst being perfectly healthy. I had to keep telling people that there was nothing wrong with me and I was going to be fine.'

The whole process was explained to Becky again and the dangers were spelled out. She was made aware that things might not turn out how she hoped and her appearance when she came round from the anaesthetic may not be the finished look. She was made aware that she could lose her nipples if they could not retain the blood supply. She was reminded about where the scarring would be after they brought the muscle forward to use as padding for the expansions ahead of the implants. Everything was spelled out to her in meticulous detail. This was really happening.

'One of the major changes over the last few years is that we are using more vertical scars', explains Becky's surgeon Andy

Baildam. Although you would not expect them to, they heal beautifully and are much more cosmetically pleasing than the horizontal scarring. They also obviate the need for scars across the upper part of the breasts or awful scaring on the cleavage.

'The first thing we did was to mark up the skin surface of the breast to measure where we would put the scars both sitting up and lying down. We used a permanent pen marker and a tape measure to do that. We try and put scars in a place where they would be least visible and we could do them to curve around the ariola at the side of the nipple and then down the mid-line of the breast. Her natural breast shape is quite high, she does not have a breast droop so we could avoid putting the scar underneath the breast, so we measured and calculated where we wanted the nipples to lie.'

What should have been a deadly serious and vitally important lesson in what would happen to her over the most precarious four and a half hours of her life was still given a lighter edge. The whole thing was being filmed.

'The hospital staff thought I was nuts. For one I had a great big film crew follow me in and most of the nurses had not been told so they all scampered away. I was taking more people into the operation room than the surgeon. Staff were amazing. From the moment I got there, people came to see if I was OK. The anaesthetist talked me through everything, the registrar came to see me, my blood pressure was taken every five minutes, but it was all good. The atmosphere was kept light, which meant there was no question of me feeling down or doubting myself.'

Becky's biggest fear was the anaesthetic. The fear was primal, once she was put under it was all out of her control and the trust was put firmly in the hands of the surgeon. It was not a fear that particularly bothered any of the medical team because it is a natural reaction to an operation and given the seriousness of what was about to happen, on the grand scale of things it was not a reason to doubt her conviction. The operation would go ahead as planned, but friends and family faced an anxious wait.

For the ITV1 crew it marked the end of a long journey as well. They had been with her from the very beginning when the genetic test results were confirmed. At the time Becky was against the idea of having them film during the actual operation, but this very soon changed as she go to know and trusted their integrity.

'At the beginning I was not sure if I wanted them in there with me, but the more I got to know them and the more good I could see the publicity was doing, I thought it was a good idea. Having them in when I was being operated on was very comforting in the end. To know there was someone there who actually cares about you. I really did believe Siobhan and the rest genuinely cared about me as filming progressed and it was lovely to know they would never let anything happen to me.'

'I have never filmed anybody I know being operated on before', confessed Siobhan. 'The first moment when they wheeled her in I did not like it at all. Ironically, it was not the operation itself that bothered me, it was that first moment when she had the anaesthetic and she was out cold with the tube in her mouth, it was quite upsetting. They put a sheet over her head so that you could only see the chest area and there was something about that I really didn't like either. I just wanted to see her face, I did not like the notion of them covering her face but the actual surgery was fascinating. I could appreciate the amazing job the surgeons were doing.'

She was now at the mercy of the surgeons.

'We made the incision and separated the fat of the skin from the breast to mobilise the whole cone of skin off the breast. We preserved little blood vessels to the nipple area because the majority of the blood comes through the breast itself, but that is what we were removing so the only supply left would have been through the skin.

Having dissected the cone of the skin from the cone of the breast we divided through the ducts behind the nipple to release it and set out to take the glandular tissue of the breast off the chest wall which is held on by a series of ligaments in front of the chest muscles. We then removed the breast cone.

'That left the muscles of the chest with the breast skin lying loosely on top of them. We made an opening under the chest muscles and went underneath using lighted endoscopic retractors that allowed us to see under the muscle to created a pocket on both sides which was of breast shape and had the same base. Having created this we inserted the tissue expanders, which are basically very expensive breast-shaped balloons with valves in them, we put those in on both sides rather like half a large pear so you put the flat side against the rib cage and the foam side facing outwards underneath the muscle.

'We then injected some saline, like you would use in an IV drip, into the tissue expanders. Each of the expanders has got two chambers so you can expand the lower part separately from the upper half. We filled those up as far as we could within safety and closed the space in the muscle, put drains in, put in sub-pectoral tubes that take local anaesthetic afterwards for post-operative comfort and care; this allowed us to reduce the amount of opiate she would need. We were then able to close up all the skin, put tape on and bandages on top of that. It was then a case of waiting for her to come round.'

Years of medical and surgical training were being put to use. The more breast tissue that could be removed, the less risk there would be of developing breast cancer. It was a procedure Wendy fought to make available, but for her the agony of seeing her daughter's chest opened up was worse than when she was on the operating table herself.

'Much worse, from Christmas until the moment she went in I was nervous and got myself a little wound up, privately of course. We always knew she was doing the right think but it is a different ball game when your baby is in there. I thought I would be awful whilst she was in surgery, but it was not as bad as I imagined. I was sat with Carl in a little room and the TV crew kept coming out to keep us updated and letting us know that it was going well. I was actually able to get on with some work, which was a good way of keeping my mind off things.'

'Both of us were very calm, which was a surprise', explained Carl. 'Wendy thought she would be pacing around the room and she wasn't. I admit I was more bored than anything else. I just wanted her to come out and see how she was and that was the one good thing about having the film crew there. I felt a bit restless throughout the operation so I went for a wander, went for a quick drive just to clear my head because it was doing me no good being in there. After the op there was that big relief, especially for Wendy that she was back and it was all over. It was just a bit weird and very hard to explain. We knew whose hands she was in and were confident that everything was going to be all right. We knew the risks but it had to be taken.'

The operation was over in a little over four hours. The surgeons were happy with how it had gone and the early word back from Siobhan, who had seen the whole process, was that Becky would most likely be delighted with the results. There were still matters that had to be attended to, for example the

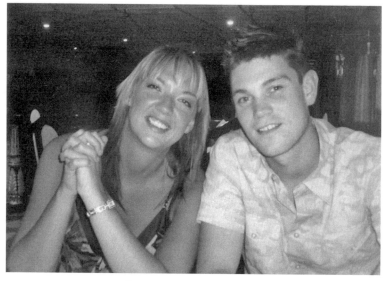

Partners – Becky and Carl

nipples had to be kept warm for 48 hours, a course of pain killers was administered and she was hooked up to a drip complete with an oxygen mask. Becky looked like she had endured an operation, but her initial feelings ensured relief amongst all those with her at that moment.

'I remember waking up with a massive smile on my face and I could hear my mum say, "Look, she's smiling", and then she started crying. They were taken out once they knew I was all right. I felt drunk from the anaesthetic, but what I remember most was that my throat really, really hurt, so I complained that I could not breath. The nurse, who was absolutely brilliant, just turned round and said I was making a hell of a lot of noise for someone who couldn't breathe. They put a pipe down your throat to help you breath during the operation, it felt so tight but it didn't hurt as much as I thought it would, I was expecting the worst pain in the world and it was not at all.

'I had bandages and tape around the nipple area and what looked like cling film wrapped around my chest so I looked down and knew they had been done. I was amazed and kept screaming at the nurse "Have you seen these?" She kept telling me to calm down but I didn't want to put my oxygen mask back on, it all seemed so new and I wanted have an explore and find out what had happened to me. Everyone was telling me to be quiet because there were other patients, I must have been a nightmare. I think if they could have put me back under at that time they would have. I was on the biggest high from the moment of coming round.'

Any concerns that she wouldn't experience the kind of relief experienced by her mother and cousin Helen were gone. She wanted to show off her new breasts to anyone who would stand still long enough, but now was not the time to get excited. She had undergone a traumatic and life-changing operation that needed to heal. The recovery time was two months. For the moment the burden of responsibility fell on friends and relatives to spread the news that the operation had been a success. It was such a relief to those who waited by the phone all day for the news that she was OK.

'My main worry was when she was in the operating theatre', recalled close friend Teresa Lomas, remembering conversations she had with Becky before the operation. 'I was on my toes all day and could not wait for the phone call to tell me she was fine. I wanted to know she had woken up because that was what she was concerned about most of all and that made me worried as well. As soon as I knew she was awake I knew she would be OK. It never really affected me until then. We talked for hours and I probably knew everything there was to know about it. I could put everybody wise and she helped me as much as I helped her in terms of preparation. It all came and went so quickly. I think she thought she was a bit of a fake afterwards because she seemed so bright.'

Carl was given the task of informing her friends. They were all told to stay away from the hospital just for that evening to ensure Becky had time to rest. It was not an easy thing to say, everybody was dying to find out how she was, what she thought, how she looked and to offer support. Wendy took it upon herself to lead the way.

'Exhaustion hit in, but I wanted everyone to leave her alone, including me. I had stayed at the hospital the night before but she needed sleep after the operation. I wanted to lead by example and leave her to recover. I did not want people piling up on her, she would still be there the following day. Everybody else could have their time with her when she felt fit enough to do so, but for that moment she needed to recover. I took some things in for her before going home. We would speak in the morning.'

If Thursday was the night before, Friday was definitely the morning after.

'On Friday morning I felt shocking, I could not even go to the toilet properly. I had antibiotics going in through my hand, a drip through my foot and two bags with drains of blood in them, so going to the toilet was a mission in itself. But to get there and not be able to go even though you need to was torture. I was sitting there for half an hour with an oxygen mask on with these two things that feel like hundred tonne weights on my front. I didn't even have any morphine because the doctor advised me against it. It was not very good at all and at one point that night they almost gave me the pain relief. The slightest movement was agony and I nearly lost all dignity but for the fact I was in so much agony.'

The feeling did not last long. The euphoria returned on Saturday, along with the realisation that, like her mother before her, breast cancer was no longer a predisposition. She was showing off her new assets to friends and family who by now were becoming more than familiar with them. Becky had pre-warned them that she might not want to show them the results of the operation because she did not know how they would look. Her fears that something would go wrong were imprinted on some of her friends. Nicky explained that she found it difficult to know exactly how to react to one of her best mates being laid up in hospital.

'It affected me more than I thought it would. We were waiting to go in with the film crew and I just could not go. I never thought I'd feel like that, but I had this vision that she would be wired up to machines and have all theses tubes sticking out of her, weak and pale. I don't know why but I made it worse in my mind and had to compose myself because I did not want her to see me upset, that would upset her. I had really not thought about it and it just overwhelmed me. I eventually took a deep breath and when I walked in she was so happy and sat upright, which really threw me. My uneasiness filtered through to her because she actually remarked on why I didn't look at her. I felt so awkward. I went a couple more times and it became easier, but it was a difficult thing for me to cope me, despite the fact she made us so aware of what was happening. I was not prepared for how it might turn out.'

Her friends rallied round and helped her with little things like putting up her hair. The procedure, though precise and complex, is still quite brutal and Becky was unable to raise her arms by herself until the Sunday. Her recovery was so swift that by Monday morning she was back on Peak FM via the telephone, talking to Sean live on air.

'It was amazing, I expected her to sound ill but she sounded so much better than I thought. The main reason we got her on the phone so early was that the listeners had been bombarding us with questions about how Becky was getting on. We kept people updated throughout Thursday but the information dried up over the weekend and people wanted to know how she was doing. It was important for us to keep them up to date and, on a personal level as friends, to keep in touch, but it was remarkable how lively she was just three days after a major operation.'

'That was fine by me', Becky recalled, 'because what was so nice was that text messages and e-mails had been sent right up to the day of the operation. I knew they had done a running commentary on Peak and that must have sounded dramatic. I wanted to come and show people I was fine, four days after the op I felt brilliant and I just wanted to say thank you to everyone as well. Rather than consent to it, I probably forced it onto Sean.'

The way Becky came through the operation amazed everyone. There was a confident air about her that was present before but quadrupled in its enthusiasm and a self-confessed new zest for life. She had grown in bra size from a 36B to a 36C, with further operations that would expand the breast envelope before another operation to put in the implants. On top of that, the dark shadow of breast cancer that had been cast over her and her mother since Wendy was 16 had been cleared. The risk of developing breast cancer had been put from 85 per cent to less than 10 per cent in four and a half hours. A death sentence had been turned into a new lease of life. Becky came out of the procedure with all guns blazing. Even her father, who had reservations about her early exposure to the realities of breast cancer and her participation in the ensuing public awareness campaign, was in agreement that it ended up working in her favour.

'As an 11 year old you are put in the limelight and it was upsetting at the time, but looking back it helped her. If there is one thing I have learnt about operations it is that modern science and technology is wonderful. She now thinks very strongly that it is good publicity to allow people the opportunity to consider the same thing and make people aware and I am all for that. No way would I want to be seen to be against that. It was brave going through with it and even braver telling everybody else about it. When she came out we took her for dinner at the pub and nobody would have known she had this operation. She had a low cut blouse on and nobody gave her a second glance and she was superb. Her confidence is right up there, more than she had before.'

'Becky is a person who really needs control,' concluded her breast nurse Lesley Thompson, 'which is one of the reasons for choosing to have her breasts removed. To wait for breast cancer to hit, you hand control over to the disease so that you have to react to it. The thing that keeps her going is being pro-active, wanting to be there first and getting it before it gets her. That has got her through everything so she was in control even from

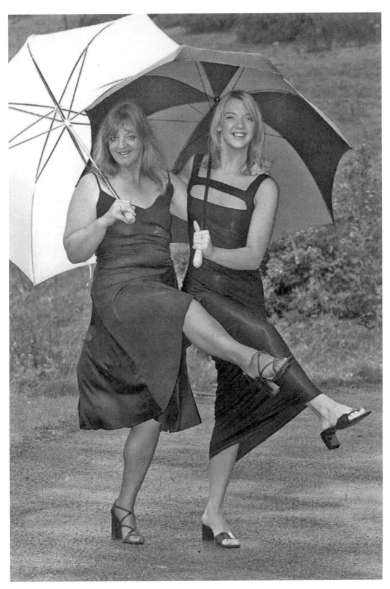

Becky left school at 18 – here with Wendy

coming round to the surgery. She asked for a sort of pain control system that she could govern, not react to somebody who came round to ask if she was in pain and give her something. Because of very simple things like that, because she has made choices all down the line; she was not going to let the surgery get her down. She has come out of it a much stronger and more confident person as a result.'

WHAT'S IT ALL ABOUT?

The decisions taken by Wendy, Vanessa, Helen and Becky were not taken lightly. Each one had a different situation to deal with a single common factor, driven by the knowledge that breast cancer would be a crucial factor in their lives. Whether choosing to have surgery or opting against it, whether to wait or take immediate action, the problem would never go away. Even if breast cancer never reared its ugly head, its presence would always be felt as a dark cloud hanging over their future. The lives of all four women have been affected by something beyond their control, yet they seized back control by virtue of Wendy's efforts to prove something could be done. Her 20-year crusade to convince GPs that breast cancer could be hereditary has enabled them to tell their stories and make sure that women in a similar situation can also take back control.

The emotion and drama that unfolded within this family mask a detailed scientific background. The fact that a person can effectively be born into breast cancer had never been taken seriously before Wendy's pioneering surgery and was frowned upon until as recently as the mid-1990s. Once the genetic fault was discovered it changed the way breast cancer was researched. Suddenly the attack was two pronged. Not only was there treatment available once the disease had taken hold, the research could also be geared towards prevention.

Everything revolves around one single gene, Breast Cancer 1, Early Onset, or BRCA1. It is a human gene that acts as a tumour suppressor, controlling the way that cells divide and multiply by reducing the probability that a particular cell will turn into a tumour. There is a second gene that acts in a similar way, BRCA2, a bigger and more complicated gene. The full extent of its function is still not known. It is a subject that Professor Gareth Evans is more than familiar with.

'If it functions properly then it looks after your DNA, checks there are no genetic errors and if it finds any errors then it helps to repair the damage along with other genes and other proteins. If, as in Becky's case, you do not have a functioning BRCA1 gene then you accumulate genetic damage in yourself and that genetic damage leads to cancer. It is a very important gene in looking after the integrity of your cells, particularly the breast and ovarian cells rather than other tissue types. Research shows that it is specifically important in tissue where oestrogen is a factor and there is a clear response of this gene to its production. It acts as a female protective mechanism to the bad effects of oestrogen production but one of the principle side effects is that women have this one in ten lifetime risk of breast cancer.'

The way the gene operates is simple. The protein produced by the gene interacts with the protein turned out through another gene, RAD51, in the nucleus of normal cells. This is how breaks in the human DNA, often caused by natural radiation or when genetic materials are exchanged for cell division, are naturally repaired. The protein made by BRCA1, BRCA2 and RAD51 play vital roles in keeping the genetic make-up stable. If there is a fault in the BRCA1 gene then the mechanism that keeps a particular cell under control fails to work. If a tumour suppressor gene such as BRCA1 mutates, the probability that a tumour will form becomes much higher.

'Essentially cancer occurs when a cell starts to grow out of control. It fails to recognise the cells around it so it begins to invade into those cells and the blood vessels and feed to other parts of the body. We are not just talking about one cell because it starts to divide and eventually create lumps and tumours. Those tumours then cause an effect by oppressing on vital structures, invading into them, destroying the function of organs as it spreads throughout the body. Unless stopped this will eventually lead to death.

'The process starts off when the genetic control of the cell goes wrong and that happens by accumulating damage in those genes that control cell growth. When those genes, or a sufficient number of them, are damaged, that cell begins to grow out of control and the worst cases see it spread around the body in the blood stream. Ideally, you are able to pick up the breast cancer before it spreads so that you have a chance of cure. It is true that chemotherapy is improving all the time, but once a cancer has spread around the body it is not an easy thing to cure.'

If a genetic mutation is found there is a serious choice to be made. Having the BRCA1 gene fault means that a woman will have up to an 85 per cent chance of getting breast cancer within her lifetime. It does not mean they have or will definitely get breast cancer; the chances of the disease hitting a person at an earlier age is not necessarily governed by carrying this mutated gene. It simply means that an affected person is one step closer to getting the disease because an important part of the gene carrier's genetic make-up is not working properly. One important aspect of a person's natural defence has been stripped away.

The genetic link was theorised in the United States in 1990 and discovered in Becky's family in 1994. Before then, linkage factors were used to determine the possibility of such a connection, which was investigated through the family tree and probability factors. By finding out who had developed or died from breast cancer using these methods, the likelihood that a certain relative or ancestor carried the gene could be determined. For example, in Wendy's case, her risk factor was at 50 per cent because it was almost certain that her mother, who died from breast cancer, was a carrier of the mutation and may have passed the gene on to Wendy. The question of whether Wendy carried the mutation was down to how the BRCA1 gene is housed in the body, within chromosome 17.

A chromosome is a thread, found in the nucleus of the cell that carries the genetic information. Each person carries two copies of chromosome 17, one from the father and one from the mother, who themselves carried two copies and so on down the generations. If Wendy's mother carried the mutated BRCA1 gene in one of her copies of chromosome 17, then there was a 50 per cent chance she would pass on the mutated version and a 50 per cent chance she would pass on the healthy one. The clinic could only put her risk of developing breast cancer at 50 per cent until they were certain she carried the gene, if that could be proven then that was when her risk factor would be put at up to 85 per cent.

Finding the gene fault was vital for Becky. If a test comes back negative and no fault is discovered then the test cannot be performed on a relative. The theory is that if there is no gene fault then the risk of it being passed down no longer remains; however, this theory is flawed. Labs in the UK do not check the whole gene. Typically 60 per cent of the gene is checked, meaning that unless a specific fault is being searched for, a negative test does not mean there is no gene fault, it just means they have not found one. A gene fault is found in two out of every ten women who are tested, that means 80 per cent of those tests come back inconclusive. Wendy chose to have the surgery without being sure because she was convinced the gene was there; however, this would not be enough for many women. The first thing to do was identify the fault.

'For reasons that remain elusive', recalled Professor Evans, 'we were not able initially to find a genetic fault in Wendy's family. Finding such a mutation is rather like finding a spelling mistake in *War and Peace*, you have to look all the way across the genetic code and sometimes the fault does not lie in the actual chapters or the writing, they occur in the binder of the book and sometimes you get chapters that go missing. In fact the genetic fault that affects Wendy's family actually lies within the binder, quite far in and it was not picked up by those initial tests. We had to go back and look at the samples several times, we had already looked at BRCA2 as well as BRCA1, so it was a matter of going back and back again until eventually we did actually find the genetic fault.'

The *War and Peace* analogy is useful when defining the process behind finding any genetic mutation. For a fault to be genetic it has to be specific to that family, in other words each family that carries a mutated BRCA1 gene has a different fault unique to that group. If a spelling mistake was to be found in *War and Peace* and that exact spelling mistake was discovered in another printing of the novel, they must have come from the same printing press. The same goes for the fault within BRCA1 and the family it is found in, so once it had been discovered, the genetic test could be developed because there was no longer any need to search the entire gene. The fault had been pinpointed and they knew where to look.

Despite the complex nature of the science behind it, and the gravity of the situation it could give rise to, the test could not be simpler. As far as the patient is concerned it is just a blood test, with a sample taken from the arm and sent to the laboratory for analysis. Of course from the scientific point of view there is more to it.

'Your red cells do not have a nucleus and contain no DNA, so you spin down the blood sample to obtain the white cells. DNA is then extracted and chopped up into pieces of a workable size. The next job is to specifically identify the part of the DNA that contains the BRCA1 or BRCA2 genes you want to work on and then analyse that particular chunk. You basically look along the sequence of the gene using a special sequencer that will give you the exact order of the four bases that make up the DNA. When a gene starts you have what we call a Starting Initiating Codon, which tells the cell to start producing a protein and then you get thousands of these nucleotides in BRCA1 and BRCA2 that eventually make up the protein. At some point the protein is formed and you get what is referred to as a Stop Codon, which stops the making of the protein. It is not the gene itself, but it produces the protein in the cells and that is what gives us the effect we are looking for. The genes are there to produce the protein, but if the genes are faulty then no functional protein is produced. This has the effect of putting that person at an increased risk because the protein and the gene are not doing the job they are made for.'

This is the point where somebody is told they have an 85 per cent chance of developing a disease that is one of the UK's biggest killers of women. Wendy, Vanessa and Becky all made their choice to have preventive surgery; Helen left it too late despite already making the choice to have surgery. As any medical professional will testify, there is no right or wrong way to approach this type of situation, it is down to a personal choice which is why all four women underwent a different decision making process. There is not just the risk of breast cancer to consider, if that was the case then the decision to go under the surgeon's knife while still fit and healthy might be easier. Becky was faced with the most difficult choice because of her age. Her breast nurse Lesley Thompson did not mince her words about what she would have to consider.

'Coming to us without breast cancer is very different from opting to undergo preventive surgery. There are big decisions and other smaller options to consider. Big options include whether or not to have the breasts removed immediately or wait until after having kids. Having surgery before means you will not be able to breastfeed and this does affect some people's decision. You can of course wait and then decide to go through with the operation at a later date, coming to us for regular surveillance. This was not an option for Becky because of what happened to Helen, but some people are willing to wait. There is also a huge option that hangs over women with a family history as to whether to have children anyway. Should they have their ovaries removed and if that is the choice they make, will they want it done in one huge operation or wait.

'Smaller options include leaving the ovaries for a while because that feels like less of a danger, but decide to have the breasts removed. In terms of other things to consider in this case, there is also the choice of whether or not to have breast reconstruction. If reconstruction is chosen then there a number of other questions to think about such as do you want to keep the nipples? Will you want to keep your own breast skin or remove everything, as it would be for someone who has actually had breast cancer. In this case the rebuild will be like the tummy tuck or the back flap for breasts. There are a lot of surgical choices that are much smaller than the bigger picture, but need just as much attention. The decision is never clear cut and should never be treated that way.'

Surgical technology is improving by the day. When Wendy had her operation, it was not possible to have reconstruction at the same time without affecting the efficiency of the operation. For Becky it was a much more viable option and cosmetically the results have also improved. The operation is currently a much more recognised and practiced procedure than when Wendy went under the knife. There is more understanding of the patient's needs. Becky's surgeon, Andy Baildam, has been amazed at the progress that is being made so rapidly.

'The expanders we have available and the implants are considerably more advanced than they were even six years ago. For example, we now have the choice of a dual-chambered expander that allows us to pump up the breast at the top and the bottom to give a more natural shape. We have a huge variety of sizes and shapes of cohesive gel implants available from a wide range of manufacturers. They are all slightly different, which means that we can choose very carefully the implants for each individual patient without having to say to people that this is the implant and if it fits then it fits, but if not then too bad. We can tailor that very carefully. The implants have changed in terms of consistency, texture and the way they feel and although they are solid, they are being manufactured to be much softer and more natural to the touch.'

Despite techniques improving by the day, surgery still has its pitfalls. Becky, Wendy and Vanessa came through their operations with the feeling of relief because their mental preparation was thorough and they felt there was no other choice to make. The threat of breast cancer is severe enough to consider a pre-emptive strike, but the implications of preventive surgery also need to be considered. Becky researched all of the options and consequences, explored every avenue in terms of the pros and cons and what could go wrong. Her breast nurse Lesley Thompson is an advocate of making absolutely certain that no stone has been left unturned.

'Women need to know exactly what they are about to let themselves in for. They need to be aware that it can be an emotional roller-coaster, because you will have this enormous relief of getting rid of the potential time bomb once the operation has been performed, but you will also have the sadness of losing your breasts. It should never be under-estimated that this is a part of the body you can have fun with, feed your children and they are intrinsic to a woman's femininity. By having a mastectomy you can never feed children and sexually they may look fantastic but you are definitely compromised because the sensation is not the same, they will no longer be sexually active. I certainly know of one woman who went through it quite young and told me it would have been better to die from breast cancer than to feel like this. She felt artificial, a case of what you see is not what you get, and the cold fact was she did not feel true to herself. Unfortunately, she had not prepared herself mentally and it is not a process that can be reversed.

'From a surgical point of view things might not go smoothly. They went well for Becky but you can get an infection, you can get bleeding, you can get some tissue that dies so you may end up with a breast that is painful, unsightly and causes you trouble. Even when it goes smoothly, there is always going to be a degree of maintenance required such as changing the implants. As you get older your body might form capsules round the implants and they may get lumpy and look strange, these breasts are not going to stay the same. They will need upgrading from time to time right through life and some people do experience difficulties.'

For many people, surgery is only the beginning. Once a tumour has been removed, the threat of it returning still remains and there is a long recovery period to ensure it does not spread any further. Becky and Wendy believed they would have to undergo a mastectomy at some point anyway, one of the deciding factors behind taking preventive surgery. By doing it on a healthy pair of breasts, the threat of breast cancer returning is no longer there because they never had it in the first place. The recovery period only took the amount of time they needed to get over the operation, unlike Helen who needed chemotherapy, radiotherapy and was put through a premature menopause. This means that four years after being diagnosed with breast cancer, despite being clear of the disease, Helen is still living with the effects. In many cases the subsequent treatment is worse than the surgery.

'Chemotherapy targets cells that are rapidly dividing,' explains Professor Evans, 'mostly by causing damage to the genes so you kill the cell off. Most chemo is more specifically damaging to tumour cells than to normal cells, but most courses do have an effect on normal cells as well. People often lose their hair because it damages the growing cells; they also feel weak and drained of energy. It is something that needs serious consideration because chemo is most definitely not a treatment to be taken lightly but we are now developing forms that are much more specifically aimed at the tumour and less harmful to the normal cells.

'Radiotherapy is the localised treatment and involves delivering a large dose of radiation, usually over a number of episodes of around 15 or 20 sessions. Women who decide not to have a mastectomy have radiotherapy for the remaining breast tissue, to ensure the tumour does not come back in the localised area. That is now the standard treatment every woman who has had cancer but not had a mastectomy will undergo. It can also treat the armpit area as well, but that is about local control; chemo is about treating it if it spreads. Radiotherapy is not going to improve or cure the cancer to the same extent as chemo because you get the same sorts of results from radiotherapy as you do from a mastectomy. It is just another means of preventing local recurrence without the more significant surgery of a mastectomy.'

Neither of these treatments is pleasant. They cause degenerative effects on the body and the patient comes away from the sessions feeling drained and exhausted to the extent that some decline further treatment in the event of a relapse. There have been a number of high profile court cases in the newspapers about patients being denied the right to potentially lifesaving drugs that could remove the need for such treatments. Professor Evans acknowledges the cases but says the treatment is not available to everyone for a reason.

'At the moment Herceptin is only licensed for treatment in women who have had breast cancer and the disease has returned. The drug company has still not put through a license, but the data we have is short term, two- to three-year follow-ups, which suggest that giving it up-front at the time of diagnosis or after the initial treatment does reduce the chances of tumour recurrence. It also potentially reduces the chances of dying of the tumour by up to 50 per cent, so it is pretty convincing evidence that perhaps it should be used in the primary setting. There is still no license, so it has to be looked at on a patient-by-patient basis, but it is very expensive. People are trying to duck out of the decision to sanction the use of a very expensive drug unless they have to and that is what all the court cases are about.

'Another treatment that has been licensed is aromatase inhibitors. This stops women producing oestrogen from their peripheries, such as the fatty tissue from the adrenal glands. Women after the menopause continue to produce oestrogen and this treatment effectively stops that happening. Unfortunately, it does not work for women who are still having periods, so the only way you can use this type of treatment is if you also switch the ovaries off, either by removing them or by using another drug that stops them working. This treatment tends to favour women who already have a family and have no plans for more children.'

The reality is that there is no miracle cure. Press reports of wonder drugs in their test stages circulate the front pages and headlines of newspapers and TV reports every month, but they never materialise. Wendy, Becky, Vanessa and Jeremy have all mentioned such reports as reasons for hope or for delaying possible surgery because the signs of a breakthrough always appear to be on the horizon. However, this is not always an outlook that produces a positive outcome.

'It can be unhelpful', admits Professor Evans, 'because it is important to make people aware that things are in the pipeline, but unfortunately these things are heralded far too early and overblown before there is good evidence that they will fulfil their potential. The likelihood is there will not be a single cure but there could be many cures. In terms of researching preventive measures, this kind of research can be counter-productive when people are being told that in a couple of years this or that could be available. People will maybe have false hope that things are going to be there for them too soon and that is when we really have to make sure people are realistic about what is going to be available.'

One of the biggest factors behind keeping breast cancer at bay has nothing to do with drugs or surgery. The way we treat our own bodies can have a major bearing on future disease; for example, a person is at an increased risk of skin cancer if they were sunburnt as a child. Dietary changes and lifestyle factors are major parts of research into the causes of breast cancer and these can be affected from an early age. Awareness is often clouded by the many reports about how eating a portion of a certain food type or even drinking a certain number of units of alcohol can change the percentage risk one way or the other. However, Professor Evans is an advocate of the theory that we can help ourselves cut that risk.

'Almost certainly the modern epidemic of obesity is going to be a huge factor and it will have its effect in two ways. Firstly bigger, fatter children will experience their periods at an earlier stage and the sooner you start your periods the greater the risk is. Certainly it massively increases a person's chances of getting breast cancer after the menopause because you continue to produce large amounts of oestrogen in the fatty tissue. We know taking hormone replacement therapy and the pill increase the risk of the disease and we need to look at alternatives in synthetic oestrogens and progesterones. Secondly, obesity tends to come at the expense of exercise and we know a good fitness regime can keep the disease from developing.

'There is some evidence to suggest that dieting for a limited period of the week can yield results and this is something we are currently working on. It is more achievable than constant dieting and we have found that in rats and mice you get more preventive effects by dieting in this way. The theory behind it is that a person would diet for three days a week, only having less than 800 calories a day, and then eat normally for the rest of the week. There is some evidence to suggest that this would be better than chronic dieting because it is extremely difficult and you deny yourself the treats that would be satisfied by the limited dieting. If you could say to yourself that you only have to diet for these three days and then give it up for the rest of the week it is a much more achievable goal.'

There is also a myth that has to be dispelled. The family tree research shows that the faulty gene can be passed down through the masculine side of the generations. Though men tend to escape the effects of the BRCA1 gene, there is a possible increase in the chance of developing prostate cancer or bowel cancer. This is not to say that men are free from the risks of breast cancer. In the 1990s there was a concerted awareness campaign to convince men to self examine for testicular cancer in the same way women do for breast cancer. There was a belief that men were failing to face up to the prospect of such a serious health issue. The same can be said of this terrible disease. Men have breast tissue, so by extension they can also develop cancerous tumours. The alarming thing is that it is not at all uncommon.

'About 300 men a year are diagnosed with breast cancer in the UK', explains Professor Evans. 'That means just under one in a thousand men will be diagnosed in their lifetime. It is a pretty reasonable number to start with and there are things that will increase the risk even more. For instance, men who are given female hormones such as oestrogen; so people who undergo sex change operations will be more at risk. They used to give oestrogen in prisons to try and calm down male patients who were too unruly, particularly in the United States, and that caused a large number of cases of breast cancer in men. Men with an extra X chromosome stand more chance of succumbing to the disease, but the biggest risk factor is a gene mutation, not as in Becky's gene but in BRCA2. This gives them a 5 to 10 per cent lifetime chance of getting it, which is a 50- to 100-fold increase risk and in line with the population risk of women.'

There is still a great deal of mystery surrounding breast cancer. There is no cure. The only guaranteed method of prevention is surgery and even that leaves a slight risk, and treatment in the event of contraction is often painful. Some people still consider elective surgery to be a drastic solution. Those who take it on believe that waiting to get the disease is even more so. At the time of writing the amount of money being spent on looking at prevention is limited. The tide is in need of turning.

A new centre is being built in Manchester, set to incorporate The Nightingale Centre, and there are hopes this will fuel a change. It will be one of the world's first research institutes that will gear its work solely towards stopping the disease before it has a chance to manifest itself. In an industry that faces competition in funding from other research projects, funding was always going to be an issue. There are a number of charities that collect for cancer research, all worthy carriers-on of the fight against the horrific effects of one of the world's biggest killers. However, there is only one that commits itself to the kind of research the new centre will provide, The Genesis Appeal.

GENESIS

Breast cancer kills one in every 30 women in the UK. Despite this shocking statistic, there is still no guaranteed way of stopping it from striking apart from preventive surgery and even this still carries a risk. Only 2 per cent of all money raised for breast cancer research is spent on prevention, the rest is spent on trying to find a cure, treatment or rehabilitation. The cost of an operation to treat the worst cases of the disease runs well into five-figure sums of money, but cost is not the issue when dealing with something that kills so many people. The human suffering that can result in contracting breast cancer would be eased considerably if it could be prevented from developing in the first place, let alone spreading. Wendy, Becky and Vanessa took this view; Helen would also agree.

There are many cancer charities that plough money into research. Of all these good causes there is only one that dedicates all of its funding to prevention and that is The Genesis Appeal. It was founded in 1996 by a surgeon called Lester Barr and a number of interested breast cancer patients, all harbouring similar concerns about why nobody was able to stop this disease from blighting their lives. The project initially had a lot of involvement with the Jewish community in Manchester, due in part to genetic links that had already been discovered by Professor Gareth Evans. The campaign was born out of a desire to raise awareness of the issue and try and develop a genetic means of preventing its onset.

'There was a group of us who felt the time had come to focus on prevention rather than cure', explains Chairman of the Appeal, Lester Barr, who is also a breast-cancer surgeon. 'There was so much research and money being spent on looking for new drugs and treatments that may never be found, but not enough looking at stopping the very thing they were trying to treat. We started the appeal to redress that balance because we felt prevention and early diagnosis might be a way forward for the next generation. Even now the perception is that scientists in a laboratory somewhere will find a magical cure, and maybe one day it will happen, but there is no sign of it anytime soon, so at the moment we need to find an alternative and that is where prevention comes in.

'Although it is true to say cure rates have risen over the last few decades because of better treatments, the number of incidents has also gone up and a lot of the good progress made through that research has been wiped out. It seemed to us we needed to look at how to reverse the rising number of women getting breast cancer and it seemed logical that stopping it striking in the first instance was an important route to look at. We felt Genesis was an important step down that path because so little money or energy was being spent in that area.'

It seemed the disease was overtaking the research. With more cases neutralising the progress of treatment, the Genesis founders were determined to take on breast cancer directly and tackle the source. The campaign is based in Manchester because of the city's links with genetic research and its association with prevention. The hospitals boast three professors who all look at different areas of research in prevention and early detection; all of whom would benefit from extra funds. The enthusiasm that was created by a common interest in seeing this horrific disease eradicated has seen the charity grow. To this date it is still the only cancer charity that puts all its money into research aimed at stopping its development.

'The majority of money we have raised has come from community fundraising groups. Some people who help us out have seen friends or loved ones affected by the disease, others may involve a group of girls or women who want to raise money through a dinner dance, coffee morning or sponsored walk. We also get help from organised groups like The Rotarians, The Lions Club and Oddfellows. If one of their members has got breast cancer they may have decided to raise money for us. The majority comes from community groups, we have not had any big grants from public companies or people leaving anything in their will, it is all individuals.'

The Genesis Appeal was gaining momentum and caught Wendy's eye. It dealt with issues close to her heart and an alliance would soon be forged that would ultimately save the very existence of the family history clinic that was so influential in her decision to undergo surgery. Following the operation and the subsequent broadcast of the Channel 4 documentary, *The Decision*, Wendy had received a great deal of media attention. The letter she received from a woman who had lost her mother and grandmother, both of whom contracted breast cancer before the age of 30, moved her to act. The woman, who lived in Nottinghamshire, was concerned she might leave her two young children without a mother, but her concern had gone unanswered by the surgeon she had seen in Nottingham. The letter distressed Wendy; it mirrored her concerns as a 16 year old, so she decided to confront the surgeon herself.

Wendy contacted the centre to explain why the woman had got in touch with her. She made it clear that this woman's mother and grandmother died young, and she was approaching the age when they had been affected by breast cancer and wanted to do something about it, or at the very least talk about it. Wendy told the surgeon that the woman did not want to put her children, who were only babies at the time, through the agony that she felt when she lost her mother. Wendy also explained her own experiences and told him how her life had taken off after taking the preventive option. The response she got shocked her.

'He was so sarcastic. He kept saying that just because I had been on TV it did not mean I knew more about the job than he did. The man continued to patronising me by calling me "My Dear" and I just thought that if that was his attitude then evidently I did know more because I understood more about how she was feeling than he did. I had made contact with him because a woman wanted to talk about preventive surgery and had the door slammed in her face; I just wanted to explain to him how I felt after having the operation. He would not entertain talking about it, told me I was being ridiculous and that was it. It made me determined to help her get a referral outside of the area so I got her one to Manchester and this guy blocked it, he would not let the Health Authority pay for it.'

It seemed the medical world was still not listening. Wendy resorted to setting up a record company and recording a single in an effort to help pay for this operation. It seemed nothing much had changed for women in her situation. However, there was another issue at hand, one that had even more serious ramifications for women with concerns that they may have a hereditary link to breast cancer. The family history clinic in Manchester was coming under threat of closure because the money from research projects was drying up. Wendy knew how important this facility was to people like her, especially in light of her experiences in dealing with the surgeon from Nottingham. The implications of its closure were unthinkable. She took her fight to the top.

'There were lots of people like me that had been with the genetic clinic. Once the funding ran out they were getting no screening or any kind of help. None of these places were getting any financial assistance because the Government was not funding genetic services. I thought it should be taken much more seriously and I was invited to meet with Baroness Cumberlidge, who was the Junior Minister for Health, a position that pretty much made her minister for women's health. I wanted her to see how important these centres were for thousand of women and they needed financial help.'

Wendy had done her homework. She presented a collection of figures that showed how places like The Nightingale Centre in Manchester were saving the Government money. Wendy's determination was to bring about another service that would once again revolutionise breast cancer research.

'I did a research project to work out how valuable genetic testing actually was to the NHS by using my family as a model. I worked out that we had saved the Government somewhere in the region of £67,000 by virtue of having a genetic test. At the time it could cost anywhere between £27,000 and £50,000 to treat somebody with terminal cancer. I compared that with how much it cost to perform preventive surgery, which was between £2,000 and £4,000. I also told her it was cheaper to treat a screen-detected tumour; in other words if they find a tumour in its early stages it was much less expensive to deal with than full-blown cancer.'

Women were on the verge of being denied potentially life-saving screening. Wendy converted this information into a language the Government finds easier to understand, cost. She hoped to ensure the continued survival of the clinic but

Baroness Cumberlidge made another suggestion that would not only benefit the clinic, but benefit thousands of women who may not even live in the area. She asked Wendy if she had considered setting up a helpline that would serve the dual purpose of giving advice to people in similar circumstances to the woman from Nottingham and give her some added clout in her lobbying. It seemed she had missed the target but hit the tree.

Wendy was offered a small grant to help start up the phone line, £10,000 for an initial three-year operation. However, there was a stumbling block. Wendy was doing this by herself and to accept the grant she had to become a registered charity, a procedure that would involve a lot of extra work. The money may well have been made available without this option because Baroness Cumberlidge would be the one to sign off the Section 64 notice. It was her suggestion so it was unlikely they would run into problems, but Wendy had a better idea, one that would also help fund genetic research and strengthen the position of the family planning clinic and the work currently being done by Professor Evans.

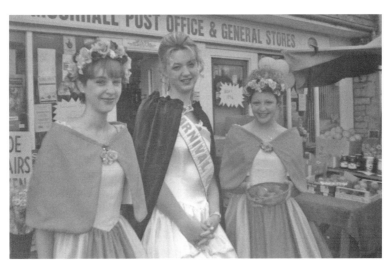

Raising funds, having fun – and winning: Bakewell Carnival Queen 1996 with Toni Thorpe (left) and Carrie Burton

The Genesis Appeal had not been going for very long, but it had established itself as a registered charity. If the helpline became part of Genesis, another arm of the appeal, Wendy would not have to go through the trouble of finding trustees because she would already be part of a registered charity. The helpline would be there for people who had concerns with hereditary breast cancer and Genesis was there to make money for research into breast cancer prevention. Both were unique yet they complemented each other perfectly; however, there was still no guarantee that the helpline would be a success. Once again it was time to enlist the help of the media.

'From the moment it was launched there was a lot of publicity because there was still a lot of interest in what I had done', explained Wendy. 'They were able to submit their reports and I could give them the helpline number to put across in their articles and radio interviews. I produced a whole batch of leaflets, gave the number to all the doctors in the UK, launched it in newspapers and magazines, everything I could think of to get the number out into the public domain. I got a list from the Department of Health that gave me the addresses of all the surgeries and sent it to every single one. It was a huge task but I made sure that every chance I got, every surgery and health clinic I could find, I gave the phone number a plug.'

The helpline was inundated from the start. The popularity still fluctuates depending on what is making the news at the time. There may be rumours of a breakthrough in treatment, a new drug or another story of courage from a breast cancer sufferer. Currently the number has three lines that are operated by Wendy and Becky from their home in Bakewell. It is still fully operational after ten years in conjunction with Genesis and was instrumental in keeping research projects alive.

'It is about giving people the options and allowing them to do whatever they want with the information that may be out there. I was also a good spokesperson for the profession, because of my close links with St Mary's Hospital and The Nightingale Centre. I could make sure that people who phoned up knew about any progress that was being made in certain areas and dispel any myths. I provided the patients with the means. I never let anybody leave without getting the referral

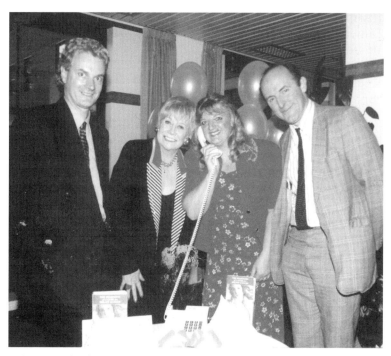

The Launch of the Help Line for Genesis: left to right: Lester Barr, Liz Dawn (Vera Duckworth in Cornotation Street), Wendy and Gareth Evans

that they wanted, whatever it took on an individual basis. Also, many genetic centres got in touch with me to talk to their service providers, the Health Authorities or Primary Care Trusts as they are now called. I did talks to them to explain why they should be funding the genetic centres along with the model that I showed to Baroness Cumberlidge.'

Wendy's determination and the clout of The Genesis Appeal had proved instrumental again. The case for prevention was gaining momentum and was beginning to be taken more seriously, but the funding was still not what it should be. Genesis was providing much needed cash and the helpline was proving that genetic research centres were vital, but the tide still had not turned, the cause needed another big push.

'Quite a bit of the funding we were getting was from Genesis', Professor Evans explains. 'There are some ongoing grants from other organisations, such as the Breast Cancer Campaign and Cancer Research UK, but it is hard to get money for research into prevention. Only 2 per cent of money nationally for cancer research is spent on prevention, although we are seeing a bit of a change in that. We hope the building of a purpose-built centre will change the focus and prove that research like this is something that needs to be considered. I am confident there will be a greater focus; certainly for raising money specifically for prevention, but also in terms of getting more money out of the existing charities that fund in this area.'

'We have raised £2 million for the centre', explains Lester Barr about the mammoth fundraising campaign Genesis has created. 'It will cost a total of £14 million pounds, but £12 million has come from the NHS. We have been working in partnership to ensure it will be an NHS facility, because we want people to know that it will be open to the public and can be accessed through your GP. We are not building a lab isolated from everyone. It will be quite unlike anything else in the country and we all believe passionately that prevention and early diagnosis will be very important for the next generation.'

The centre helps display the strength of conviction within the charity. To start with an achievable aim of raising awareness, to pioneering a prevention centre in ten years is an incredible feat. It is making a difference that goes beyond awareness. It is providing people like Professor Evans with the means to look for a way to stop breast cancer killing people and about saving lives and families. His role within the centre will be to lead research into high-risk situations, such as those people who carry the BRCA1 fault, and to develop prevention projects. It is a project that is growing in force.

'The research will include a wide range of projects, including anything that might reduce the risk of developing breast cancer from lifestyle factors, diet and weight, through to drugs which we hope to develop, including existing drugs used in trials. We will also look at the surgical side as to which techniques offer a better chance of protection, right across the board of existing therapies.

'It is on track at the moment to be finished in early 2007 and we hope to move in by July of that year. The facilities will include office space for researchers, a physiology lab and a gym, because part of our lifestyle approach will be health related. We are going to have rooms to see people for consultations and we will be looking at bone density, which is an issue for people with breast cancer, particularly when taking anti-oestrogen tablets that could limit bone growth and we need

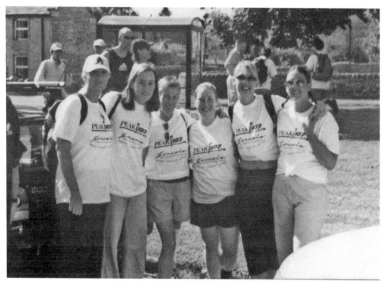

The White Peak Walk – in aid of funding for the Genesis Appeal in 2003 left to right: Teresa Lomas, Louise Hamilton, Chris and Katie Noweill, Becky and Susanne Baker

to be able to monitor that. There is a whole range of things that we want to put into the prevention centre to push things forward.

'Hopefully there will be a great deal of demand for the centre, but you can never be sure until it is up and running just how popular it will be. We hope that women will be only too keen to come up and be involved. We are looking forward to this being a major project for the future. The focus will be on what we can achieve that will not be at the expense of that individual's lifestyle; we do not want to stop breast cancer on the one hand but make life intolerable on the other. It should see the funding increase and help to bring in the best researchers to study in this area and I am confident we will begin make a difference across all fronts.'

What could be problematic is the use of case studies. The BRCA1 gene increases the probability of somebody getting breast cancer, but does not guarantee the disease will strike. This makes research into prevention difficult to prove because any positive outcome in tests performed may be affected by the 15 per cent chance that a genetically pre-disposed person may not have contracted it anyway. Research projects at the centre need to be chosen carefully and require a lot of help from potential patients.

'We can make certain predictions as to the likelihood of whether someone will develop breast cancer, based on family history and other risk factors, so we can gather groups of people at increased risk. We then need to look at putting them into studies and matching them to see whether certain treatments reduce the risk of them getting the disease. The more extreme examples are those who carry the gene mutations and have a high risk of BRCA1, so we can do a certain amount of prediction and matching, but it does mean you need large numbers to prove that something works. The ideal trial is one that randomises what you do, so you do not give everyone the same treatment, otherwise you have no way of knowing whether it is making a difference. The problem is that people with a very high risk are difficult to randomise because they know there is a 50 per cent chance that they are not being given the treatment and that's very difficult for them to consider. It is also difficult to us because we are potentially denying them life-saving treatment'

The centre will see involvement from Europe and there are already people on the scientific board from across Europe and the United States. With enough collaboration with interested parties overseas, there is the potential for the centre to become international. These are exciting times for the pioneers of genetic research and the grand opening will be a proud moment for the founders of Genesis, as well as for Wendy and Becky, whose work on the helpline kept the family history clinic operating.

The tide is beginning to change. The new centre has the potential to come up with a way of preventing breast cancer; possibly even a cure that does not involve the relatively crude method of breast removal. The decision Becky made has brought the issue to a new, younger generation who are now becoming aware that breast cancer is not necessarily something that comes later in life. The UK looks set to become a world leader in cancer-related genetic research, thanks in no small part to the likes of Wendy and Becky who crusaded to get their concerns about hereditary causes heard. The future seems a lot brighter, but there is still plenty to do and more hurdles to overcome.

THE BIG PICTURE

Becky has been extremely fortunate. Her choice seems outrageous but the factors behind it reveal a young woman desperate to escape the clutches of a disease that killed 12,696 people in the UK in 2003, according to the latest figures from Cancer Research UK. Breast cancer is the third most deadly cancer in the country behind lung and bowel, accounting for a twelfth of all deaths, frightening figures for a disease that will mainly target just half of the population. Becky worried about breast cancer but never had to deal with its effects, only the threat. It kills a third of the people who contract it and leaves the rest with the concern that it could return.

The disease has many symptoms that are not always cancerous. Lumpiness around the breast can become more obvious just before a period, cysts can develop that are nothing more than fluid or it could be diagnosed as fibroadenoma, a condition common in younger women caused by a harmless collection of glandular tissue. Other symptoms such as inverted nipples, dimpling and a change in breast size can be put down to other, much less serious conditions. Despite these possibilities, the fact remains that it could be breast cancer and early detection is one of the major factors towards increasing the chance of survival. If in any doubt the advice would always be to visit a doctor.

Breast cancer is very complex. There is no single cause and even carrying a gene mutation such as BRCA1 only accounts for 5 per cent of cases. It does not discriminate between UK regions, class, race or fitness levels, the only variants appear to be age and gender. The disease mainly strikes women between 40 and 65; however, the number of deaths has fallen slightly since the late 1980s. In 1994 deaths among women were closer to 14,500, meaning that on average more than 1,000 more breast cancer sufferers have been saved over the last decade. Some of this is down to early detection, but Professor Karol Sikora, Professor of Cancer Medicine at Imperial College, Hammersmith Hospital,

London, hails advancements in the medical world as a major reason.

'Surgery is much simpler and a lot more can be done as an out-patient. Radiotherapy has become more precise and one can avoid problems to the nerves, lungs and spinal chord because of better computerisation and planning of the radiotherapy. With chemotherapy it is all about trying to tailor the treatments to the individual and the most recent advance is trying to look at the genetic pattern of the tumour using RNA expresser chips. You can look at tumours to which you would usually assign aggressive chemotherapy, but the gene chip may tell you it is not going to become that severe. You can reduce the aggression of the chemotherapy and still get the same end result.'

Surgery is still the primary cure for breast cancer. Every person undergoes some form of surgery, even at the diagnosis stage because a tissue sample is needed from a biopsy. It is after diagnosis that the situation becomes more complicated.

'There are many different types of breast cancer recognised down the microscope', explains Professor Sikora. 'No two breast cancers behave in the same way, every one is individual because the molecular changes that led to that cancer differ enormously. Although we can recognise broad patterns, the molecular background will almost certainly pre-define the outcome, so you have very aggressive cancers and ones that are much less so. There are cancers that respond to hormone drugs and cancers that do not, ones that respond to drugs and ones that prevail. As medicines and technologies advance we have got better at sub-classifying the disease, tailoring and individualising the treatment to make sure that it is the right treatment for the right patient.

'Most women get the whole tumour removed with a free margin of at least half a centimetre around it. If the breast is going to be conserved then the normal recommendation is to give radiotherapy to the affected breast and that prevents the disease coming back locally without the need for a mastectomy. That is what we call conservative management. The third way of treating it is with drugs and there are two main classes, the first is the hormones for tumours that are responsive and have the oestrogen receptor; there are a set of hormonal treatments available depending on whether a woman is pre- or post-menopausal. Then there is chemotherapy with drugs that stop cancer cells dividing.'

Most treatments have side effects. Hormonal drugs have fewer, although they do stop periods in women. It is the chemotherapy that can have a devastating impact. Courses vary depending on the variant used and that in turn depends on the relative aggression of the breast cancer. The more invasive the tumour, the harsher the course of treatment, especially if it has spread to the lymph nodes. There is a course that has been launched in the United States and is being tested in this country called adjuvant chemotherapy. Professor Sikora is an advocate because it runs along the lines of current research geared towards personalising the treatment for specific cases.

'It can be used for both breast and colon cancer and is a treatment given immediately after surgery. It is a risk benefit analysis so you can see the percentage gain you get in terms of survival by doing particular interventions. We know that when a cancer is just a few cells in diameter, drugs are more likely to have an effect and can get to the tumour with more ease. The best time to give chemotherapy to someone who is at a high risk of developing the spread of the disease is immediately after the operation, within a few weeks, that is adjuvant chemotherapy. It comes from the Latin verb *adjuvo*, which means to throw, so you are literally throwing the drugs in at the time when the chances are high that the cells have already spread, but you can reduce the risk of them growing.'

Professor Michael Baum is Professor Emeritus of Surgery at University College London and spent 40 years working within the NHS. He recognises the significant strides that have been made in treating women, a move that has seen cure rates rise and mortality rates fall. It is not just in the success of the treatments that progress has been made, but also in the emphasis placed on the welfare of the patient.

'Patients with positive breast cancers were started off on tamoxifen, but these have been replaced by aromatase inhibitors. For the 70 per cent of women whose tumours are sensitive to hormones, these treatments have improved enormously. They are kinder than chemotherapy and have been associated with a 30 per cent fall in mortality. There are still plenty of cases that will require chemotherapy, but nobody is compelled to take that course of action, although we are talking about major improvements in the chances of long-term survival. Even though the treatments are toxic, they are associated with a 25 per cent improvement in survival and most of the side effects can be dealt with over a short timescale; however, I do not want to minimise it. Chemotherapy is tough, but it is of limited duration.'

Professor Baum performed one of the first ever mastectomies on a woman with BRCA1. The procedure was done in the early 1990s at The Royal Marsden, before the gene had been discovered. He has overseen advancements in the care of cancer patients, but the strides taken in treatment is secondary to the work done to improve surgical techniques.

'The biggest revolution was way back when I started in this speciality. All women had a radical mastectomy before a group of us became utterly unconvinced that this in itself cured breast cancer. A number of clinical trials were started up in the United States, Italy and the UK, comparing the radical mastectomy with new techniques in breast-conserving surgery. These were started up in the early 1970s and by the early 1980s there was sufficient evidence to convince anyone with an open mind that breast-conserving treatments were equal in outcome to radical mastectomies and much kinder on the patient. There are still about 30 per cent of patients who cannot avoid a mastectomy with the best will in the world. For those people reconstruction and plastic surgery has advanced in leaps and bounds. The majority of women will end up with a breast and will be able to wear normal clothes, which is a big advance.'

The operation to remove a cancerous tumour is similar to the one performed on Becky. In her case, all of the breast tissue was removed to prevent a potential tumour having anywhere to grow. In the case of a breast cancer patient, a tumour will be removed along with some of the breast tissue to ensure that it does not return.

'Becky's operation, using tissue expanders is more commonly used after breast cancer', explains Lester Barr, a surgeon in Manchester and founder of The Genesis Appeal. 'In breast cancer cases it is more common to only have one side done and in order to get a more natural feeling breast, more symmetrical with the normal breast, we often recommend the LD flap. We simply take some tissue from the back and use it to rebuild the breast tissue. It is a piece of tissue usually known as the love handle, in other words we grab a handful of tissue that we use to rebuild the breast. A similar procedure is the TRAM flap and a modification known as a DIEP flap. The lower abdominal fat is used to rebuild the breast area, it is very similar to the tummy tuck and the scar in your stomach is much the same.

'Reconstruction has been one of the big advances in breast-care surgery in the last 15 years. Until the techniques came along you had to put up with having just an ordinary mastectomy and then putting something in your bra, the advances have made a huge difference to thousands of lives. These operations are relatively recent and have been rolled out to surgeons across the country. Not everybody has had access to it immediately and it has taken time for it to be available across the UK. In theory most women who are having or have had a mastectomy should have a surgeon relatively local to them to carry out that sort of operation.'

There are concerns about a postcode lottery. An audit inquiry last year revealed that the uptake of Herceptin in Dorset was 90 per cent among eligible women, whereas in Derby that percentage was less than 5 per cent. The recent licensing of such a drug may alter that, but it does little to alter the perception that the level of care a patient receives can depend on where they live. Mortality rates do not back that up, but there are moves to try and bring about equality in treatment.

'The quality of care does vary as well as drug prescribing', admits Professor Sikora. 'What is hidden and is much more difficult to quantify is the level of expertise that is available in different areas and how that differs. Over the next few years the policy is to offer people four different choices, but at the moment it is just for surgery. It will eventually move to cancer and I think people will get the choice again. Ironically, in the good old days of the NHS there was no problem, a GP could refer you anywhere, these days it is all cost accounting.'

A centre built in London could change that further. It is being constructed at the Harley Street Clinic and will be networked with five NHS cancer centres. Professor Sikora, who is involved in the London Cancer Group that is behind the scheme, hopes it will revolutionise the way treatment is delivered across the country.

'Britain's health service is changing so we must look at ways to bring the expertise of the independent sector into the National Health Service. The idea is to create a cancer network that embraces the private sector as well as the public sector. The technology is exactly the same but it could bring all sorts of networks, created to deliver care, much closer to people's homes. A big cancer centre may have 20 associated cancer centres out in the suburbs, so women with breast cancer could have radiotherapy locally. They would not have to come to a centre in the middle of a city and yet have the same quality of care, supervised in the same way as if they were in a large centre.

'The Department of Health is looking into building 100 more cancer centres in the grounds of local hospitals. The day centres would be able to change with the times, offer radiotherapy and chemotherapy in a much more convenient way. If you look at how retail shopping works, everybody has moved out of town to these shopping centres and the same principle could apply to medical care, especially something like cancer that may require frequent visits. The whole experience would become less frantic and the level of care more fluid.'

'We are a relatively small country', explains Professor Baum, 'and compared with the travel problems we would face in places like USA and Australia, women do not have such obstacles. There is no question that travelling backwards and forwards for radiotherapy on a daily basis and chemotherapy on a three-weekly basis is exhausting and it would be much nicer for women to be able to have these treatments closer to home. It is easier with chemo because you are just carrying drugs and syringes, but there is no way at present to stop women from travelling to the radiotherapy centres daily for six weeks.'

Professor Baum, however, is involved in clinical trials to revolutionise radiotherapy. Intra-operative radiotherapy involves placing a special probe into the breast area where the tumour was removed during surgery; it produces a radiation beam that covers the surrounding breast tissue. Theoretically this tissue will be unaffected by the cancer and will nullify the need for out-patients to undergo a course of radiotherapy that could run every day for a six-week period. The treatment will last for half an hour, after which the surgery to remove the tumour will continue. The treatment is currently in an experimental stage and can only be used on women who do not have a mastectomy. It is an indication of how far technology has come in terms of reducing the physical impact of breast cancer treatment.

Recovery from treatment can vary dramatically. In some situations a long course of chemotherapy can delay the second reconstruction, an option that is left up to the individual. It also depends on the severity of the cancer in the first instance and the timing of detection. The true nightmare for a breast cancer patient in remission is if it returns. The longer a patient is cancer-free after the operation, the more the risk of its return is reduced. By its very nature, a return can never be ruled out.

'It has the ability to spread to other parts of the body', explains Lester Barr. 'That is why the whole subject is so emotive, because not everybody is cured and it can come back or spread somewhere else. These are cells growing out of the normal control mechanisms, so we may not be able to stop them growing in a particular place or stop them returning from somewhere else. If that happens then that is what we call secondary cancer and that is precisely why breast cancer is such a dangerous disease. Like other cancers, that is what it does and that fear will always remain in the back of somebody's mind.

'In terms of what to do if it does return, that depends on the individual situation. Sometimes the person may need an operation to remove a second tumour but sometimes the cancer may come back in the lung or liver or a place where you cannot operate. You would then need chemotherapy or radio-therapy treatment to deal with the secondary breast cancer.'

It is a disease that has no sense of timing. There is no effective way of predicting exactly when it will strike beyond the hit and miss reliability of a mammogram. As a consequence there may be other factors to consider. Wendy and Becky were both able to choose when to have their mastectomies; Helen was booked in within two weeks of being diagnosed. The sooner a cancer is operated on, the better the chances of survival and the kinder the subsequent treatment. This can throw up some truly devastating decisions that could seriously affect the way the patient views life itself.

'If a patient is pregnant at the time of diagnosis,' explains Lester Barr, 'then we sometimes have some very difficult decisions to make. If it happens early in the pregnancy then a decision about whether or not to carry out a termination will have to be considered. The woman may need chemotherapy that could not be administered and delaying treatment until after the child was born could jeopardise its effectiveness. If it is diagnosed later in pregnancy then it might be possible to induce the child early. Surgery during the middle or last three months is possible because of the advances made in anaesthetics. The surgery is not internal in the same way as a heart or a bowel operation so most women will cope with it extremely well.'

People are affected as much psychologically as physically. They must face up to the fact that they have a one in three chance of dying and undergo surgery knowing that a long and difficult period of recovery lies ahead. A woman's femininity will be compromised; they may also lose their hair during treatment. After all that there is an uncertain future with the constant concern that it could return and the process would have to be repeated. Doctors and GPs have the clinical expertise to deal with the tumour but a human angle needs to be injected to ease the distress that will manifest along with the tumour. A breast cancer victim will often have support from family and friends, but sometimes this is not enough.

Breast cancer can be tremendously isolating. When Helen Cauldwell spoke about her time at The Christie in Manchester. She compared her experience with the other patients as being like a self-help group. In many cases sufferers need to talk to people going through the same experience, believing nobody else will understand what they are going through. A system of support is vital. As well as pioneering surgical reforms and researching kinder forms of treatment for post-operative women, Professor Baum can lay claim to initiating the current support system. It dates back to the 1970s and came from his desire to implement a more considerate form of surgery.

'It goes back to when I first took an interest in breast cancer. I realised there were a lot of unmet needs for diagnosed women because it comes as a double whammy. Not only is it a threat to their life but it is also a threat to their feminine identity. The breast is one of the paramount icons of femininity and these women were experiencing enormous levels of distress coming to terms with losing them. None of us were adequately trained to deal with the emotional aspect because we were taught that our foremost responsibility was to diagnose and cure. It convinced me that we needed additional agencies to treat these women.

'I came up with what I thought was the simplest of ideas, to take a nurse off the ward, train her to know as much about breast cancer as I did, but also to learn about counselling. The nurse would know about all the practical aspects such as support that we were not very good with, things like prostheses, bras, how to dress, how to regain self-confidence, relationships with husbands and children and it seemed like a niche market. We identified this void and set up a programme of training such nurses and now it is so well established, you cannot have a breast unit without having specialist nurses as counsellors. I don't mind very much, but my contribution to this was forgotten a long time ago.'

His legacy certainly lives on. The support network for breast cancer patients, their families and carers, has grown to become an integral part of the entire treatment process. From the moment a person is diagnosed a team of psychologists, counsellors and trained nurses are made available to talk to about the myriad options and what may happen to them. The realisation within the health service that this is not just a physical, but also a mental issue, has revolutionised breast cancer care.

'There is a lot more support than there ever used to be', explains Dr Emma Pennery, a Nurse Consultant with Breast Cancer Care based in West London. 'Within hospital settings the key source of support comes from breast-care nurses who provide both emotional support and information. They allow patients to be able to go through things at a slower pace than they possibly might with a doctor, to revisit things on the telephone afterwards as well. Checking out what is going on and understanding treatments and results is crucial and enormously re-assuring.'

Technology has pushed the support network forward. The internet has helped to put people in touch and there are a number of chat rooms and websites that do that. It is another means of allowing sufferers to find out more about treatment by discovering how others fared by using it. Breast Cancer Care has an after nurse e-mail service that allows sufferers the chance to get a response to a question at any time of the day or night. Chat rooms and internet services also bring together vulnerable groups who may feel even more isolated because they do not fall into an age group or gender associated most frequently associated with breast cancer.

'You can talk to people across the country. You do not have to be geographically near to them or well enough to travel and these support groups often bring together slightly more unique people. Younger victims of breast cancer are more of a minority. They might not meet anyone in the hospital where they are being treated that they can relate to. By joining in these support groups, they can talk to six or seven other people in their age group across the UK and they can share their experiences. It is not always about emotional support, it is sometimes about talking to someone who is, or has been in the same situation and appearing normal.'

'I think there are about 4 million sites if you go on the internet', remarks Professor Baum. 'There are some very good ones, such as Breast Cancer Care, Breakthrough and Cancer Research UK, which are audited and have good scientific content, but there are so many it can become confusing. It is important to refer to books and medical advice that will provide audited lists of reasonable websites, but I am not entirely convinced it makes up for the personal touch. The communication skill of the doctor is the single most important contribution to the psychological welfare of women based on empirical data. If patients are asked specifically then they will say that it is all very nice having this additional support, but they would rather have it first and foremost from the doctor.'

Of course there is one type of patient who will feel even more isolated. Breast cancer is frequently referred to as one of the biggest killers of women in the UK. A lot of the after care treatment and advances made in prostheses are geared towards reconstruction of the breast and how this affects the woman's femininity and well being. What it also does is alienate the 300 men in the UK who are unfortunate enough to be diagnosed with breast cancer, a disease that common perception labels feminine.

'It is very important that we try and talk about people with breast cancer rather than women', explains Doctor Pennery. 'The difficulty men face is that they are such a minority and may not meet another man being treated at the same time. They can feel enormously isolated and even slightly embarrassed. Breast Cancer Care launched a booklet dedicated to men because of disturbing stories about very inappropriate information, post surgery, on things like bras and periods. The booklet is absolutely man-specific and a much more sensitive way of dealing with it and the feedback has been really positive. We also offer training about men with breast cancer to health professionals, so that if they do only come across it infrequently, they can provide better care.'

Studies suggest men want hard facts rather than support. Similar studies also suggest women prefer to talk to people and share experiences, two very different ways of coming to terms with and coping with a shattering disease. There are many cancer charities that have websites with helplines, links to chat rooms, information about treatments, new breakthroughs and statistics. The Cancer Research UK site also has links to specialist clothes shops that cater specifically for women who have had mastectomies or reconstructive surgery, as well as details of related events by region. The internet has given people access to a wide range of information, but Professor

Baum is a firm believer that the system of personal support has got it right.

'The main thing is the recognition that breast cancer is a very complex subject, it demands many disciplines working closely together. When I came into the subject, the surgeon was the only man, and it was always a man, treating breast cancer. Now we are working within a federal group of specialists with a common interest, surgeons, radiotherapists, medical oncologists, clinical nurse specialists, pathologists, radiologists, and we all work in these multi-disciplinary teams. We have been encouraged to give up general surgery and to focus on this very complicated and sensitive area so that right now in this country, everybody is within easy reach of such specialist multi-centre and multi-disciplinary teams.'

But there is still work to be done. Patient care amongst breast cancer sufferers is still advancing and as Professor Baum was keen to emphasise, treatments such as chemotherapy are tough. Just as support services have catered to the emotional and mental side of the care process, technical advances continue to have effects on patient welfare. Worldwide statistics show more than a million people are diagnosed with breast cancer every year, but they vary wildly from country to country. Incidents in the United States, France and Denmark are in the region of 80 to 100 cases per 100,000 women, as many as five times higher than those in China, Zimbabwe and India. Migrants from low-risk countries suffer an increased risk if they move to a high-risk country. This all adds credence to the theory that environment, diet and medical side effects are significant factors in causality.

'Diet is very closely related,' agrees Professor Sikora, 'but the research is very complicated and the studies are relatively dull. You have to collect huge amounts of information from a lot of people and it can be seriously flawed. Nobody can really remember what they ate yesterday let alone last week so it can be unreliable and is a very difficult study to do. The other problem with breast cancer is that the way lifestyle factors impinge on risk is probably through the hormonal make up. There may not be a direct link between diet and breast cancer. It could be more to with how it affects the hormone cycle, not necessarily about what is being eaten or how their life is being lived. That is very complex because of the sheer number of factors involved.'

Research is ongoing to reverse this trend. The battle to prevent the disease goes hand in hand with better treatment for those already afflicted and there is reason to be hopeful that techniques will improve as much in the next years as they have in the last.

'Women will always need mastectomies but there may be alternatives to surgery in breast cancer cases', explains Lester Barr. 'Rather than having the lump cut out we may be able to destroy it, but for those that do require surgery, the techniques are still improving. We place as much emphasis now on the cosmetic side of things than we did ten years ago and it is important to us that women retain their self-esteem, confidence and body image. In the past, many women who had a mastectomy were unable to look at themselves in the mirror, never showed their body to their partner or husband or may never have had sex again. A mastectomy can be hugely devastating from a psychological point of view and can really interfere with your sex life. By putting more emphasis on a good cosmetic outcome, we hope the quality of life will not be affected and that is how things stand.'

'We are in a very, very exciting period in the evolution of the treatment and prevention of breast cancer', agrees Professor Baum. 'We are learning so much about the molecular nature of cancer that treatments are going to be specifically tailored to the tumour. Herceptin is one of the first of these beautifully elegant, biologically engineered treatments that complements the humanity of current breast cancer care. With the specialisation and establishment of psycho-social oncology running in parallel, we have the compassionate human arm of medicine and the scientific and molecular arm, both increasing in strength.'

'I think we have got there in spite of Government interference. It frustrates me that all of the progress made by researchers, surgeons and medical experts is entirely thanks to those doctors and nurses. All of the organisation and re-organisation has contributed nothing to the welfare of women with breast cancer. We have often had to raise the money ourselves through charity. It is almost considered a joke to say trust me I'm a doctor, but that is how it is. I would rather trust my colleagues than any politician when dealing with the lives of women with breast cancer.'

Advances are being made all the time. Surgery and the treatment of breast cancer is still tough but the tide has turned in favour of the patient's comfort and care. As research continues to plug away at the root causes of this dilapidating disease, it also continues to provide better treatment and care. Mortality rates are falling but not fast enough and until prevention, an absolute cause or a cure for this disease is found, women will continue to associate breast cancer with death.

TOMORROW

Becky can now look to the future with a sense of optimism. The operation has left her with a risk of breast cancer reduced from 85 per cent to less than the general population. The expansion has boosted her bra size from a 36B to a 36D; the only thing left is to replace them with the implants. Concerns that the surgeon and breast nurse may have harboured about negative reactions to the operation can be laid to rest as Becky looks forward to living without fear. A positive outlook was part of the solution, but a sense of realism also prevailed, born from a lifetime of living with the disease without feeling its physical effects. Now that has been lifted and replaced by freedom, there is a lot for Becky to explore.

'It was such an emotional ride rather than a physical one, especially the run up to the operation, which tired me out. I had enough of talking about it and just wanted it done; now it is, I feel fantastic. Since coming out of hospital it has been a constant high, the anaesthetic probably didn't help at first, one minute I would be high as a kite, the next minute asleep, tired during the week but fine at weekends. I never thought the operation would change me but it has. I feel more confident and I was no shrinking violet before the op so that was unexpected. I have a new lease of life that I thought had run out, but things I used to find important are not so important anymore. If someone tells me my bum is too big I don't care, as long as I'm all right and everyone else is happy, then so am I.'

Becky returned to work amid a blaze of publicity. While she was recovering the fundraising continued unabated, using the surgery to bring in more money for Genesis and raise awareness in the way Wendy had before. Her co-presenter on Peak FM, Sean Goldsmith, launched a scheme that was initially created as something to talk about in Becky's absence; however, such was her popularity among the listeners and the extent to which her plight had captured people's imagination, it caught on.

'We did the "Bra for Becky" appeal', recalled Sean, 'where we asked listeners to send in a bra with a donation. It may have been a listener who suggested it to start with, I can't remember, but it helped keep Becky alive in the show and kept the talk about breast cancer and Genesis going. It was amazing; I expected perhaps 100 bras with a pound in each one, possibly £200 was the best I had hoped for. In the end we got £7,000, which is amazing, and with Becky's popularity it was still in people's minds at the time. People still responded as they followed the story through her recovery and now there is no real story to follow. She has done all she needs to do.'

There were still plenty of ideas on the breast theme. Becky is still determined to carry on the fundraising for the people who helped to rid her from the shackles of breast cancer. Still using the media world to her advantage she organised a 'Bra Tour' across Chesterfield. The idea was to persuade men and women to pay a certain amount of money for a ticket that would allow them to have a free drink at several venues across the town centre. Each reveller had to have a bra visible about their person and the fun, which took place on Sunday 28 May 2006, was open to men and women. It was an important event because it was raising the awareness of a serious issue among the groups who were least conscious of the facts, young women and young men. The event raised £3,000 in one night and Becky is keen to carry on the work they started.

'Ever since I came out of hospital and been back on the radio, the fundraising side of it has gone mental. People are raising money left right and centre and I do try to get involved as much as I can. Obviously, there is only so much that I can do, only so many places I can be, but I will continue to raise money for Genesis. There is my mum's helpline as well, which is funded by Genesis, and that is something very close to our hearts and we think is very much needed. If mum did not run the helpline then there would be no support system for people in the same situation. OK, there are other breast cancer helplines, but none that deal with hereditary breast cancer, so that is something that I will continue to help mum with as much as I possibly can.'

The final piece of the awareness jigsaw for Becky was the ITV documentary. It was screened at 11.00pm on Tuesday 6

June 2006 amid a great deal of publicity. Becky was on GMTV and *fivenews* on the day of the screening to try and drum up support; it was even named "pick of the day" in some TV listings and women's magazines. There was some initial concern over the timing of the programme, it was on very late and Becky wanted it to be screened earlier. For contractual reasons there was a limited amount of publicity she could do before the show was aired and it was scheduled to be shown earlier in the year. However, the programme did not fail to disappoint and it allowed Becky a unique view of herself that few people ever see.

'It was weird seeing myself being operated on, it did not look like me. The strangest part was seeing myself under the anaesthetic because my eyelids are taped shut and there was a tube coming out of my mouth. It is quite detailed but not over the top and the graphic part, the surgery, is left until right at the end but it is very well explained. There were parts where I was surprised because I had never seen what the expanders looked like and Andy Baildam, my surgeon, talks it through well and it is fascinating. In some respects I wanted them to move out of the way because I could not see enough.

'I am extremely happy with the finished programme and it was everything I wanted it to be. They had completed 50 hours of filming and I had no idea how it would be put together or what the outcome would be so I was a bit nervous. There are places where I thought my face looked fat or that I did not look very good, but to be honest, it did not matter because the content is so good. I'm so pleased with it because it is an emotional story, it can make you cry but because it's so uplifting rather than upsetting and that was what I wanted to see come through.'

'Everybody who has seen it has been moved', said producer Siobhan Sinnerton with a sense of pride. 'When you talk about breast cancer, particularly when a 23-year-old woman is being told that they have to have their breasts removed, one would naturally expect that it was going to be quite harrowing but it's not. There are parts of it that are sad but overall it comes across as a very uplifting, moving, inspirational film and that is not something I could have predicted at the outset. By putting up the helpline numbers after the programme, along with other websites and fact sheets, we hope it will get a response. Any woman who has not thought about a family connection, not been aware of a genetic link and goes to get tested, if even one person can be prevented from going through the horror of breast cancer, I would be delighted.'

One and a half million people tuned in to watch. It was the highest rated programme for that time slot on that night across the terrestrial and multi-channel platforms. The response was sensational. Hundreds of e-mails and texts poured into ITV and Peak FM, the helpline was also inundated with calls as the message the producers tried to get across reached its intended audience.

'They have been inundated with goodwill', confirmed Siobhan. 'The level of activity on the helpline was phenomenal, with lots of women about to undergo the same process phoning up to say they felt completely differently about it. It makes the whole thing seem worthwhile because that was what we set out to do. To try and educate and demystify the whole process. If a significant number of people benefited from that then I am delighted. Our duty office at ITV was inundated with calls and e-mails just to say how inspirational Becky was and people that were going through all sorts of personal trials and tribulations saying her experience and attitude put it all in perspective for them. I think a lot of people also hope to make money for Genesis.

'One guy wrote in, a middle-aged businessman packing for a trip, who said he just happened to catch the start of the programme and was totally engrossed for an hour and thought she was so inspirational. He was moved by her experience and wanted to donate £1,500 to Genesis. That is amazing because it was not someone who even wanted to watch the programme, but it made a connection and he was so moved by her personality and story. To know that we got through to people like that was so pleasing.'

It struck a chord with the general public. Here is a selection of e-mails sent to Becky through her Peak FM address that displays the level of feeling her story attracted.

I was diagnosed with the BRCA2 gene a year and a half ago and have been burying my head in the sand ever since, saying I'd wait until I was 30 before I thought about surgery. After seeing you go through it. I've realise I'm being selfish about the whole thing. I have a wee boy who is 8 years old and I owe it to him to go through with the surgery. My own mum died from breast cancer at 31, so I should really have had no second thoughts about having it done in the first place. You have given me the boot up the backside that I needed, so thanks again.

Jacqueline, Glasgow

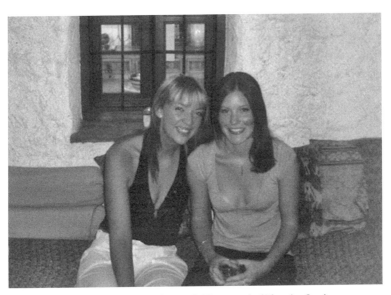

Glad it's over – Becky and Clare on holiday in Spain

I watched your documentary and felt the need to contact you as I too am BRCA1 positive. I am currently trying to work through in my mind about having my breasts removed. I'm 32 and discovered the gene in our family four years ago. I often feel isolated as being a young woman with something like this to face seems very rare and your documentary struck many chords with me.... So many people either don't understand, as they think cancer does not strike young people or they think I'm over the top!!! You voiced many of my thoughts and it is nice to know other women feel the same as me. Thank you for making me no longer feel so isolated.

Orienne, Huddersfield

Hi Becky, just wanted to say well done for the documentary. Your mum's story 11 years ago was how I found out I had a future and I had my surgery in December 2004. Like you I have a similar family history. Your film was very positive and I hope it improves the attitudes I have encountered, particularly with dating – men are not necessarily breast orientated but they are frightened of getting involved with somebody who carries a dodgy gene .... I am still glad I saved my life.

Kay, Northampton

Life with the TV crew gave Becky a taste for the medium. When she joined Peak FM it was always her ambition to move into television and her experience may hold the key to opportunities in the future. She has already appeared in the background of such ITV series as 'Crossroads' and 'Peak Practice', as well as in front of the tough judges on 'Pop Idol', although she did not make the final TV cut. With the documentary now out of the way, she is free from contractual obligations to pursue any avenue of her choice.

'My career has always been focused on that type of thing but I have been at Peak FM for four and a half years now. I am more than happy, absolutely love it here, but I'm only 24 and I have to go for as much as I possibly can to feel that I have fulfilled everything I want to. If it was not for the operation, I would still be just flowing along, but because of what I have been exposed to I realise that life is too short and it can be turned off just like that. It makes you think that you have to get yourself sorted and get a move on. It has given me the kick up the backside that I needed. It has also opened up a number of opportunities for me that otherwise would not have been there.'

One of the bigger problems facing Becky's career choice is choosing exactly what to do. Everybody wants to be famous, but to have ambition without direction is not a recipe for success. It is a cynical world and Becky's anxious not to be known as the girl who had her breasts cut off. She has her foundations in presenting and has interviewed the likes of Liberty X, Sir Cliff Richard, Meat Loaf and Ronan Keating. This is a path she would like to follow.

'The showbiz side of things is something I would like to get into. My dream job would be the showbiz presenter on "GMTV". I think Davina McCall is fantastic and I look up to her a lot as someone I greatly admire. I have done theatre since I was very young and singing was something I wanted to do more than anything. I got to the stage where I told myself to give it up, but it is something I would like to resurrect and if I can raise money for charity at the same time then so much the better.'

'She has worked so hard with her show reel', confirmed friend Nicky Bacon. 'She would love to present and would be a natural for it. She is not scared of anyone or anything and is not afraid to be in front of a camera or on the radio. If she can just make a go of it, she has taken every opportunity so far and hopefully the TV appearances she will get from the ITV programme will count towards that. At the moment she is happy with life on the radio but wants to advance that. She has been through so much and come out the other side a stronger person.'

However, the media world is a harsh one. Hard work and enthusiasm is not always enough and Becky knows that fact, having worked within the radio industry for just short of half a decade. Her health choices have worked out for her, but Sean knows that her career choices need to be just as well informed.

'I would use Holly Vallance as an example. She was in a soap opera and had a number one song, she was a massive profile, a good-looking girl but I cannot see her ever making another record. She will probably never have that kind of profile again so if Holly Vallance fails, I fear that if things work quickly for Becky and she gets a lot of TV work it could all end in five weeks. If she has to make a decision between Peak FM and TV work, it could all fall flat very quickly and I would hate her to make a decision like that and fail. She said to me recently she hopes it will never come to that, but it is a fickle business and she really wants it so badly. I hope she does not make a decision that turns out to be very wrong.'

Becky still needs to go under the knife. The reconstruction is not finished because the expanders need to be taken out to give her a more natural look. The procedure is not particularly severe.

'We will need a second operation but it will be a small one', explains her surgeon Andy Baildam. 'The expanders are only temporary and we will need to put in what are likely to be high molecular weight cohesive gel silicone implants. They are given what the manufacturers call a lifetime guarantee, but she will need further surgery to replace them. It is likely that her shape will alter or there may be some firming up of the implants, she can also get what is called a capsule forming around the implants and that can make the breast become quite hard. Although the rate of that is very low with these modern implants it can still happen and there is maybe a 5 to 6 per cent risk of that. Because the implants are under muscle, the action of the normal working muscle can push them slightly sideways or downwards. If that happens we may need to reposition them through surgery.'

The dark cloud of cancer can still cast its shadow. Breast cancer may have been beaten, but the BRCA1 gene still has another trick up its sleeve. Ovarian cancer is still a threat and the gene brings about a similar increase in probability of this form of the disease as it does with cancer of the breast. Similarly, there is no cure so another trip to the surgeon will have to be made at some point in the future.

'The risks of getting ovarian cancer are very similar to breast cancer', explains Professor Gareth Evans. 'Having children is protective, a late menopause is against you because the more you ovulate and the more cycles you have, the more risk there is. The main difference is that the combined contraceptive pill is protective against ovarian cancer. Ten years will halve the lifetime risk of getting the disease. The pill actually increases the risk of breast cancer; the risk factors are the same apart from the pill usage.'

In terms of body impact, the operation is more extreme than the mastectomy. The process involves removing the ovaries and the fallopian tubes through keyhole surgery, being careful not to leave any tissue behind because the risk would still remain. The reason it is so drastic and why Becky will not consider this for the foreseeable future is that women are put into an early menopause. This reduces the risk of breast cancer, which is not a factor in Becky's decision any more, the bad side is that, aside from the onset of menopausal symptoms

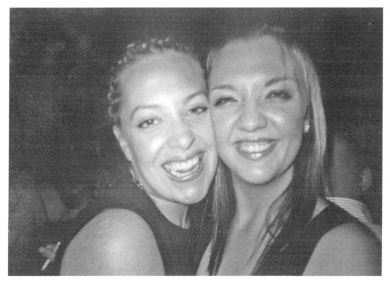

Nicola Bacon and Becky – friends matter

such as hot flushes and mood swings, the patient can no longer have children.

'I am very conscious of that and it probably worries me more than the breast cancer. It has been suggested that I have the operation at around 35 so there is a while to go yet; I have got time to have children. People are often surprised when I say I want to have kids and I know another woman with the very same gene who was frightened to death. She did not want a girl and was thankful she had two boys. To me it doesn't matter, because it would not become an issue for another 30 years or so.

Things do progress and even if no cure is found then I hope my children will get something out of what myself and my mum went through. It has definitely made me who I am, so I would not think twice about becoming a mum. It never even crossed my mind until people asked me about it.'

There has been a development that could change the nature of gene testing. There are concerns that the test to discover if a person has a genetic fault could become unavailable. The problem does not lie in the technology or the willingness of the medical profession to deal with the consequences. The problem could arise as a consequence of its discovery all those years ago in the United States. It is a familiar tale in a world obsessed by profit and loss; the reason boils down to money.

'The BRCA1 gene was originally identified in an American lab', explains Professor Evans. 'Scientists in Salt Lake City made the breakthrough and the company is now known as Myriad Genetics. They put in a patent application to protect the uses of the gene and were given permission to put in a very extensive application, allowing pretty much anything that flowed from the gene to be subject to royalties or licensing for exclusive use to Myriad. The good news is that the patent was thrown out of the European Court and at the moment Myriad does not hold similar restrictive rights in our part of the world. The bad news is that they still do in North America and are enforcing that patent in terms of the genetic test. The upshot of that is that nobody else in America is allowed to offer genetic tests.'

Lawyers set about trying to make the gene patentable. The concern for researchers is that if the use of the gene is restricted, it would make it very difficult to develop any cure that could be put on the market because a fee would have to be paid. It would not stop research, because that can be done behind closed doors; the problems would begin as soon as any breakthrough was made.

'Really it was a spurious argument because you would not have to patent the gene itself. Whatever was developed from the gene would almost certainly be patentable in its own right and would be a much more worthy patent than putting one on something that is actually part of natural existence.'

It is a big argument that still rages. Huge amounts of money were spent on getting a similar patent through the European Parliament, who passed the directive. In theory it meant the genes that were patented in the United States could be patented in Europe, although the initial outlook looks good. Researchers are confident that the laws will be interpreted more strongly against the patenting of genes in Europe as they were in the United States, but the jury is still out. The BRCA1 patent was thrown out on a technicality rather than an issue of whether it was morally or legally right. There is still the possibility that the use of the gene could be limited and the fight goes on.

'I do not think the patent will affect any of the research and certainly will not have a negative impact on any of the work we do within the walls of the new centre in Manchester. As long as you use something purely for research, whether you use patented genes or not, it really does not matter. You can get round the patent if it is used just on research, the main issue is that the whole saga could be a blight on developing preventive treatments or curative treatments based on the gene itself because you would then have to pay. It might also stop you informing patients of their genetic test results. It is a waiting game at the moment but we have no way of knowing which way it will go.'

From a patient point of view the outlook may look uncertain. Treatments such as Herceptin and, until very recently, aromatase inhibitors, were initially withdrawn from patients because of the cost to the health services. If the same were to happen to the issuing of genetic test results then a similar situation could ensue, especially considering the low level of money spent on preventive research. For the moment the research and genetic testing goes on and Professor Evans sees no reason to change the approach to his work.

'I think in terms of where genetic research is going, it is really more of the same and a case of finding out exactly what the gene does. We also need to work out what the long-term consequences are of carrying it and what we can do to reduce the risks of disease. There is the issue of discovering which families of BRCA1 and BRCA2 will help you identify other families that have to be hereditary, that do not have faults in either gene and hopefully we will come up with other definitive genes. That could also help us understand why some BRCA1 and BRCA2 families have a higher risk of breast cancer than others.'

It is a project that coincides with Wendy's research. She has carried on the sort of research that helped track down Vanessa and traced the gene all the way back to Elizabeth Land in 1780. It is a big project, but one that has the backing of the family history clinic.

'With Gareth the project is two pronged', Wendy explains. 'One part is to look at all the families in Manchester and Birmingham that have a genetic fault, taking notes from every person and their first-degree relative. We then look at what form of cancer they have and how old they were when they were diagnosed to get an idea of what the life expectancy is of a person who has that particular gene fault The other side is to create family trees to link up different families. In one case I have gone back about 200 years to the same area and hope to find the link. Once I have completed that project, I would like to do family trees in a more general fashion to see if there might be a young death and get the death certificate to see if there is any kind of family history of disease. I could try and date it back to 1837, the year the civil register started, and see if there is anything that has remained in the family.'

One trick that is proving elusive is correction of the gene fault. Gene therapy has worked in some instances and some research has already been made into trying to get the BRCA1 gene to function again. If the gene's function is to regulate the cycle of cell division, controlling the growth of cells, there could be some way of recreating this function in the event of a gene fault. Unfortunately, it is not as simple as reparation.

'What we will be looking at eventually', explains Professor Evans, 'is finding small molecules that do the job of the BRCA1 gene. It has been developed for a number of other conditions and there is a whole breed of new treatments that essentially do just that. The only way you can make the BRCA1 gene work properly again is to actually repair it. That is almost impossible to do in every breast or ovarian cell. Gene therapy, as in repairing or putting back the good copy of the gene, is being looked at but up until now has proven very difficult to achieve outside conditions where you can get at the tissue concerned and particularly where you can use bone marrow. This means that it has worked well in circumstances where we can get at the bone marrow, change the gene and put it back in again. We do think, however, that it is unlikely to work for a cancer condition so what we can work towards is finding small molecules or drugs that do the trick.'

He will be getting extra help in funding the centre. With Becky's story inspiring an influx of calls at the helpline, Genesis is expanding its horizons as well. Having already contributed £ 2 million to the cause the charity is stepping up its campaign with a new wave of fundraising. Carrying on with its grass roots ventures, they have initiated plans to directly fund the workings of the centre.

'We have completed our target in terms of raising money for the centre,' explains Lester Barr, 'but our focus must now change. Whereas for the last six years it has been about the bricks and mortar, from now on we want to support the people working in the building. We are looking to develop a team that will allow people to sponsor one of our research workers in a similar way that people can sponsor a child in Africa. A donor will have a personal link to someone who is directly responsible for the research work and we hope that will have an appeal.'

This is not to say grass roots work will be forgotten. The charity still has plans to back a number of ventures that continue to chip away at the problem while celebrating the human triumph behind many stories of the disease.

'We tend to leave it to people's imagination in terms of actual ideas, so we do not start the year with a list of things to do. One thing we are doing this year is a breast cancer fashion show where all the models have had breast cancer. It is great fun and very moving because it is about real people who have battled the disease and want to make a statement that, despite going through the pain of the disease, they are still beautiful people. It is important, not only as a fundraising idea, but it makes that statement about how it can devastate your life but you can take control of your own life and not let it beat you.'

With the introduction of the prevention centre in Manchester, the future in terms of research looks bright. Becky has taken over the mantle from her mother in many respects in terms of raising awareness of breast cancer and proving that there is an alternative to waiting for it to strike. Her age and glamorous appearance belie the worries she has carried for so many years and is an example to a younger generation that cancer is never something that happens to other people.

'I am a normal 24-year-old girl and have always considered myself to be normal, with an ordinary childhood and average upbringing but with an exceptional background. If I want to go out and have a drink with my friends I do not want people looking at me as if I shouldn't in case it triggers breast cancer. I want to be normal like everyone else, and for me the operation was my opportunity to have a normal life without breast cancer constantly looming over me. I am trying to make something good out of a situation that is not good. I hope that by making my story public, I can help other women who find that they have the breast cancer gene.'

Like any other woman, Becky has ambitions. Whether it is to break into TV or stay at Peak FM, resurrect a promising showjumping career or have another go at singing on stage. The one part of her life that has remained constant throughout the genetic test and the operation is the unwavering support from her family and boyfriend Carl. Their relationship has blossomed over the six years that they have been together and they can look forward to the future, although any plans of marriage have been put on the back burner by both of them.

'God no, we don't talk about marriage yet. I'm too young and we enjoy having a laugh with our friends as much as each other. This year has been hectic and we agreed to leave things for the time being, but next year we do have plans to buy a house, which is frightening. We are happy and will continue to be so.'

'We haven't spoken seriously about anything like marriage', agrees Carl. 'We have been through so much over the last couple of years, now that is out of the way we can live a little

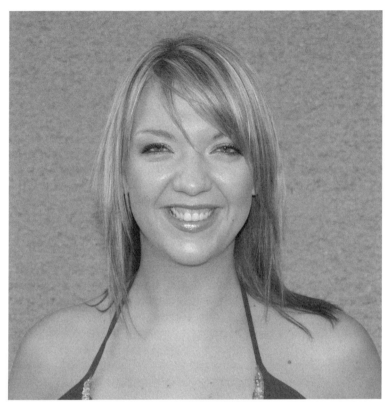

Becky today

and then think about settling down if we think it is the right time. We have to buy a house first so that will be the next big thing. The only definite thing that has been mentioned was that she would have to sort out the downstairs department, because the same gene affects ovaries as well. She needs to have kids before she reaches 35, according to the doctor's advice, so as far as the future goes we just leave it at that and see what happens.'

Becky feels that the experience has changed her for the better. She has spoken of her new zest for life, a renewed optimism over her life choices, the publicity for herself and for cancer awareness and the burden of concern lifted from her shoulders. She bears no hostility to the gene that could have caused her so much pain, instead regarding it as just another part that makes her the person she is now. It is this attitude that allows her to think about having children without concern for passing on the gene. Adopting that stance also equipped her with the self-esteem to regard the loss of her breasts with the view that there is more to her now than there was before. The one word so many people have described her as is brave, that is not how Becky sees it.

'I don't think it was brave, I just think it was sensible. I think I would have been silly if I opted against having the whole operation. My feeling was that if I did not do this and I ended up getting cancer I would be a very selfish person, because I have seen how it can affect people. It does not just affect the person who suffers from it, friends and family suffer too and I was given a chance to prevent all that. There are not many women out there who can say they had a choice. I have got my pick of the best surgeons in the country, possibly the world, who will look after me for the rest of my life. I would be selfish if I did not have this done and that was my feeling throughout the whole thing. One in nine women out there have never had a choice and I am sure if they did, they would have done exactly the same as me.'

ACKNOWLEDGEMENTS

There are a lot of people I would like to thank, without whom writing this book would have been a much less enjoyable experience. First of all, my fiancée Jenny, put up with my endless hours at the computer, furnishing me with cups of tea and keeping me going throughout. I hope our children have her patience and not mine! Thanks go also to Mary and Mike, Jenny's mum and stepfather, for the occasional use of their computer and to my mum and dad for believing I could do this and encouraging me all the way. I am also very grateful to my friends Matt and Louise, Jim and Rachel, Seb, Jenny and Mark, as well as Jenny's friends for distracting me enough to enjoy the odd beer now and then.

Special thanks go to David for giving me the opportunity to write this with what was a tremendous leap of faith, and to Mark, who trawled through my first draft with a fine tooth-comb and taught me that it is more important to know where you are wrong than where you are right. I am extremely grateful to Clive, whose guidance and advice taught me more in the last three months than I have learnt since college, also to Naz and the rest at Peak FM for the time off and the use of resources to conduct interviews.

To those who contributed, I owe a massive thank you, in particular Helen for speaking so candidly and her two dogs for making me so welcome. I also owe a huge debt of gratitude to Gareth for going out of his way to fit me in whenever I needed to speak to him, and for his patience during interviews that ran well over time. My thanks go too to Vanessa for her help in allowing me to better understand a complicated family tree, to Lester and everyone at the Genesis Appeal for their kind help, and to Andy for going out of his way during an incredibly punishing schedule – a tough man to track down.

None of this would have been possible without the co-operation and help of Becky and Wendy – Wendy for trusting me to tell her and Becky's story, for her enthusiasm spurred me on and she was always available to talk, and to help with the family tree.

Finally, to Becky, who asked me to help with the notes that led to this opportunity and for never tiring of me asking the same questions over and over; I will be eternally grateful. She is a good friend and work colleague – we must do it again some time!   *ST*

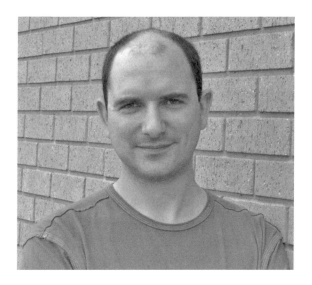

Simon Towers was born in Keighley in 1976 and lives in Sheffield with his fiancee, Jenny. His first writing experience was a puzzle page for the Ghostbusters magazine at primary school. With an honours degree in the history of art, design and film from the University of Northumbria, he took a post-graduate diploma in bi-media journalism at All Saints College, Leeds, worked at Stray FM, joined Hallam FM and is now co-writer and producer of Peak FM's weekly sports review; he created their DVD review section. This is his first book

Kirsty – Angel of Courage by Susie Mathis
The little girl who touched everyone's hearts

'Her attitude is amazing and her courage is extraordinary' –
a remarkable little girl'

Chris Tarrant

Kirsty Howard was born in 1995 – and given six weeks to live. She is the only British child born with her heart back to front. After nine major operations, she is still here, her future still grimly uncertain.

She has met Royalty, pop stars, sporting heroes and Hollywood actors. She has the support of the Prime Minister and across the nation. She has touched the hearts of millions here and overseas.

Kirsty's Appeal for Francis House, the only Manchester Hospice for terminally ill children, seeks £5 million, and is almost there.

This is Kirsty's story in words and pictures.

Medavia Publishing
an imprint of Boltneck Publications of Bristol

Medavia is a major media agency and Medavia Publishing brings people in the present and facts about the past into print.